The Diabetic Foot

Editor

FABIAN KRAUSE

FOOT AND ANKLE CLINICS

www.foot.theclinics.com

Consulting Editor
CESAR DE CESAR NETTO

September 2022 • Volume 27 • Number 3

ELSEVIER

1600 John F. Kennedy Boulevard • Suite 1800 • Philadelphia, Pennsylvania, 19103-2899

http://www.theclinics.com

FOOT AND ANKLE CLINICS Volume 27, Number 3
September 2022 ISSN 1083-7515, ISBN-978-0-323-91983-8

Editor: Megan Ashdown
Developmental Editor: Arlene B. Campos

Foot and Ankle Clinics (ISSN 1083-7515) is published quarterly by Elsevier, Inc., 360 Park Avenue South, New York, NY 10010-1710. Months of issue are March, June, September, and December. Periodicals postage paid at New York, NY, and additional mailing offices. Subscription price per year is $351.00 (US individuals), $763.00 (US institutions), $100.00 (US students), $378.00 (Canadian individuals), $786.00 (Canadian institutions), $100.00 (Canadian students), $489.00 (international individuals), $786.00 (international institutions), and $215.00 (international students). To receive student/resident rate, orders must be accompanied by name of affiliated institution, date of term, and the *signature* of program/residency coordinator on institution letterhead. Orders will be billed at individual rate until proof of status is received. Foreign air speed delivery is included in all *Clinics* subscription prices. All prices are subject to change without notice. **POSTMASTER:** Send address changes to *Foot and Ankle Clinics*, Elsevier Health Sciences Division, Subscription Customer Service, 3251 Riverport Lane, Maryland Heights, MO 63043. **Customer Service: 1-800-654-2452 (US and Canada). From outside of the United States and Canada, call 314-447-8871. Fax: 314-447-8029. E-mail: JournalsCustomerService-usa@ elsevier.com (for print support); JournalsOnlineSupport-usa@elsevier.com (for online support).**

Reprints. For copies of 100 or more, of articles in this publication, please contact the Commercial Reprints Department, Elsevier Inc., 360 Park Avenue South, New York, NY 10010-1710. Tel.: 212-633-3874; Fax: 212-633-3820; E-mail: reprints@elsevier.com.

Contributors

CONSULTING EDITOR

CESAR DE CESAR NETTO, MD, PhD
Assistant Professor, Director of the Orthopedic Functional Research Laboratory (OFIRL), Department of Orthopedics and Rehabilitation, University of Iowa, Iowa City, Iowa, USA

EDITOR

FABIAN KRAUSE, MD
Associate Professor, Department of Orthopaedic Surgery, Inselspital, University of Berne, Berne, Switzerland

AUTHORS

HELEN ANWANDER, MD
Department of Orthopaedic Surgery and Traumatology, Inselspital, Bern University Hospital, University of Bern, Switzerland

MARTIN C. BERLI, MD, PD
Deputy Head, Division of Technical Orthopedics, Department of Orthopaedic Surgery, Balgrist University Hospital, Zurich, Switzerland

THOMAS BÖNI, MD
Head, Division of Technical and Neuroorthopaedics, Department of Orthopaedic Surgery, Balgrist University Hospital, Zürich, Switzerland

CARLO BIZ, MD
Associate Professor, Orthopedics and Orthopedic Oncology, Department of Surgery, Oncology and Gastroenterology DiSCOG, University of Padova, Padova, Italy; Minimally Invasive Foot and Ankle Society (MIFAS by GRECMIP), Negrevergne, Merignac, France

KEIVAN DANESHVAR, MD
Head of MSK Imaging, Department of Diagnostic, Interventional and Pediatric Radiology, Inselspital, Bern University Hospital, University of Bern, Bern, Switzerland

CHUI JIA FARN, MD
Department of Orthopedic Surgery, Inselspital, University of Berne, Berne, Switzerland; Department of Orthopedic Surgery, National Taiwan University Hospital, Taipei, Taiwan

THOMAS HESTER, BSc(Hons), MBBS, MSc, FRCS(Tr&Orth)
King's College Hospital, London, United Kingdom

CHOON CHIET HONG, MBBS, FRCSEd
Department of Orthopaedic Surgery, National University Hospital, Singapore

MATTHEW J. JOHNSON, DPM
Assistant Professor of Orthopaedic Surgery, The University of Texas Southwestern Medical Center, Dallas, Texas, USA

VENU KAVARTHAPU, FRCS(Tr&Orth)
Associate Professor, King's College Hospital, London, United Kingdom, University of Southern Denmark, Denmark

CHRISTOPHE KURZE, MD
Department of Orthopedic Surgery, Inselspital, University of Berne, Berne, Switzerland

OLIVER MICHELSSON, MD
Orthopeadic Surgeon, Foot and Ankle Surgeon, Terveystalo Helsinki, Univeristy Hospital of Helsinki, Helsinki, Finland

ROSLYN MILLER, FRCS Tr&Orth, MBChB, BscMed Sci
Professor, NHS Lanarkshire Universities Hospitals, Lanarkshire, Glasgow Caledonian University, Glasgow, Scotland, United Kingdom; Foot and Ankle Service Lead, Department of Orthopaedics, Hairmyres University Hospital, East Kilbride, Glasgow, United Kingdom

NGWE PHYO, FRCS (Trauma and Ortho)
Consultant Orthopaedic Surgeon, Department of Trauma and Orthopaedics, Frimley Park Hospital, Frimley Health NHS Foundation Trust, Surrey, United Kingdom

STEFAN RAMMELT, MD, PhD
University Center for Orthopaedics Trauma and Plastic Surgery, University Hospital Carl Gustav Carus at the TU Dresden, Dresden, Germany

KATHERINE M. RASPOVIC, DPM
Associate Professor of Orthopaedic Surgery, The University of Texas Southwestern Medical Center, Dallas, Texas, USA

PIETRO RUGGIERI, MD, PhD
Full Professor, Orthopedics and Orthopedic Oncology, Department of Surgery, Oncology and Gastroenterology DiSCOG, University of Padova, Padova, Italy

JAMES SIOW, MD
Department of Orthopedic Surgery, Woodlands Health, Singapore; Department of Orthopedic Surgery, Inselspital, University of Berne, Berne, Switzerland

ERKKI TUKIAINEN, MD, PhD
Professor of Plastic Surgery, Orthopeadic Surgeon, Plastic Surgeon, Department of Plastic Surgery, Univeristy Hospital of Helsinki, Helsinki, Finland

FELIX W.A. WAIBEL, MD
Consultant, Division of Technical and Neuroorthopaedics, Department of Orthopaedic Surgery, Balgrist University Hospital, Zürich, Switzerland

ALEXANDER WEE, FRCS (Trauma and Ortho)
Consultant Orthopaedic Surgeon, Department of Trauma and Orthopaedics, Frimley Park Hospital, Frimley Health NHS Foundation Trust, Surrey, United Kingdom

DANE K. WUKICH, MD
Professor and Chair, Department of Orthopaedic Surgery, University of Texas Southwestern Medical Center, Dallas, Texas, USA

Editorial Advisory Board

Contents

Foreword: Shooting Star: A Tribute to Alexej Barg   xiii

Cesar de Cesar Netto

Preface: Dear Foot and Ankle Surgeons!   xv

Fabian Krause

Diagnostic Imaging of Diabetic Foot Disorders   513

Keivan Daneshvar and Helen Anwander

Plain, weight-bearing radiography is the preferred first-line imaging. Dependent on the suspected pathology, further imaging is indicated. In a soft tissue infection, an abscess has to be excluded, for example, with ultrasound. Osteomyelitis has a typical triad including osteolysis, periosteal reaction, and bone destruction in radiography, but signs are often delayed. MRI is the gold standard for diagnosis of osteomyelitis with high intensity in T2-weighted and STIR images and intermediate to decreased reticulated hazy intensity in T1-weighted images. In comparison, bone marrow edema is also bright on the T2-weighted image but the T1-weighted image has a confluent low intensity.

The Interdisciplinary Approach: Preventive and Therapeutic Strategies for Diabetic Foot Ulcers   529

Christophe Kurze, Chui Jia Farn, and James Siow

The appropriate treatment of the common diabetic foot ulcers (DFUs) in diabetic patients demands enormous human, organizational and financial resources that are finite. Interdisciplinary teams of medical and surgical specialists, as well as allied health professionals, can help to reduce the consumption of these resources, optimize treatment, and prevent DFUs. They consist primarily of vascular surgeons, endocrinologists, and orthopedic foot and ankle surgeons and are closely supported when required by infectious diseases specialists, plastic surgeons, wound care specialist nurses, podiatrists, and orthotists. A timely interdisciplinary team review in each clinic session decreases the number of hospital visits for the oftentimes-handicapped diabetic patients significantly. The interdisciplinary team clinic setup has also been shown to reduce the risk of amputations, length of hospital staz and mortality rates.

Distal Metatarsal Osteotomies for Chronic Plantar Diabetic Foot Ulcers   545

Carlo Biz and Pietro Ruggieri

In more than 30 years of scientific literature (1986–2021), the few published studies on the management of CPDFUs by DMOs showed satisfactory clinical and radiographic outcomes. Although these reports were all case series, their data suggest that DMOs, performed at a different level of the distal metatarsal bones, are an effective surgical treatment option for achieving rapid healing of CPDFUs and preventing their recurrence after balancing the pressures in diabetic forefeet. Hence, DMOs can be a valid alternative treatment method also for CPDFUs with chronic infection, ulcers penetrating deep structures, and even ulcers with osteomyelitis at the metatarsophalangeal level.

NEMISIS: Neuropathic Minimally Invasive Surgeries. Charcot Midfoot Reconstruction, Surgical Technique, Pearls and Pitfalls   567

Roslyn Miller

The last decade has seen a significant development in early surgical intervention for patients with or at risk of ulceration owing to deformity resulting from the sequalae of diabetic foot disease. Midfoot Charcot neuroarthropathy is the most common deformity; its correction is enabled by specialized surgical implants designed to maintain surgical corrections. There has also been an increasing number of orthopedic foot and ankle surgeons, with a specific interest in diabetic foot disease who provide early surgical correction in patients identified as high risk. Minimally invasive surgery using percutaneous incisions completes the triumvirate, facilitating earlier surgical intervention to decrease reulcerations.

Etiology, Epidemiology, and Outcomes of Managing Charcot Arthropathy   583

Thomas Hester and Venu Kavarthapu

Surgical intervention for Charcot arthropathy is becoming more common; this is driven by an increased prevalence, better understanding of the cause, identifying patient risk factors that influence outcomes, and how to best optimize these. This article aims to summarize the cause of Charcot, look at the factors that influence the outcomes, and the financial cost of managing what is a very challenging condition.

Nonoperative Treatment of Charcot Neuro-osteoarthropathy   595

Felix W.A. Waibel and Thomas Böni

Conservative treatment of Charcot neuro-osteoarthropathy (CN) aims to retain a stable, plantigrade, and ulcer-free foot, or to prevent progression of an already existing deformity. CN is treated with offloading in a total contact cast as long as CN activity is present. Transition to inactive CN is monitored by the resolution of clinical activity signs and by resolution of bony edema in MRI. Fitting of orthopedic depth insoles, orthopedic shoes, or ankle-foot orthosis should follow immediately after offloading has ended to prevent CN reactivation or ulcer development.

Managing Acute Fore- and Midfoot Fractures in Patients with Diabetes   617

Choon Chiet Hong and Stefan Rammelt

Few is investigated about the management of acute fore- and midfoot injuries in diabetics. With well controlled diabetes, indications and techniques are similar to non-diabetics. With poorly controlled diabetes, medical optimization should be exercised. Stable internal fixation in case of surgical treatment and prolonged offloading independent of the choice of treatment are advised. With manifest Charcot neuroarthropathy, the goal is to achieve a plantigrade, stable foot that is infection- and ulcer-free and ambulant with orthopaedic shoes. If operative treatment is chosen, the concept of superconstructs in combination with prolonged protection in a well-padded total contact cast is applied.

Managing Acute Ankle and Hindfoot Fracture in Diabetic Patients   639

Ngwe Phyo and Alexander Wee

The management of ankle fractures in the diabetic population requires special attention as the risks of injury or treatment-related complications are high. Thorough review of clinical history and detailed assessment provide the treating surgeons with key information to guide treatment pathway. Vigilance is required when opting for nonoperative treatment in undisplaced stable ankle fractures in patients with peripheral neuropathy. The presence of critical ischemia in injured limb demands vascular consultation and ultimately, an intervention before surgical fixation of ankle fracture. An extended period of immobilization is one of the key principles in the management of ankle fracture patients with diabetes.

Limb Salvage in Severe Diabetic Foot Infection   655

Dane K. Wukich, Matthew J. Johnson, and Katherine M. Raspovic

Severe diabetic foot infections (DFI) are both limb threatening and life threatening and associated with negative impact on health-related quality of life. Most severe DFIs require surgical intervention, and the goal of treatment should be preservation of limb function in addition to eradication of infection. Minor amputations are required in approximately 40% and major amputations in approximately 20% of patients. Significant risk factors for lower extremity amputation included male gender, smoking, previous amputation, osteomyelitis, peripheral artery disease, retinopathy, severe infections, gangrene, neuroischemic diabetic foot infections, leukocytosis, positive wound cultures, and isolation of gram-negative bacteria.

Minor Forefoot Amputations in Patients with Diabetic Foot Ulcers   671

Oliver Michelsson and Erkki Tukiainen

The prevalence of diabetes mellitus, particularly type 2 diabetes, is increasing worldwide. Also, the incidence of both lower limb revascularizations and amputations is increasing. We have less transtibial amputations due to improved diabetes care, but also due to modern treatments, vascular surgery, and development of plastic surgery. With well-planned minor amputations, more limbs can be saved. Minor limb-saving amputations are preferred especially to older diabetes patients, because they have a high-risk contralateral amputations. Losing both limbs causes major problems for patients and their life, risk for lifetime ward is high.

Mid- and Hindfoot Amputations in Diabetic Patients   687

Martin C. Berli

Several surgical options exist to avoid or at least to delay a below-the-knee amputation (BKA). These are the so-called mid- or hindfoot amputations. They are a valuable treatment option in order to maintain the ability to ambulate without major auxiliary means (eg, a prosthesis). Hence, these

amputations allow the patients to maintain a certain autonomy. The acceptance of these amputations is significantly higher than a BKA, as the body
image is less disturbed. The complication rate in hindfoot amputations in
diabetic patients is high due to the comorbidities, in particular peripheral
arterial disease and polyneuropathy.

FOOT AND ANKLE CLINICS

FORTHCOMING ISSUES

December 2022
Managing Challenging Deformities with Arthrodesis of the Foot and Ankle
Manuel Monteagudo, *Editor*

MARCH 2023
Applied Translational Research in Foot and Ankle Surgery
Don Anderson, *Editor*

JUNE 2023
Advanced Imaging in Foot and Ankle
Jan Fritz, *Editor*

RECENT ISSUES

JUNE 2022
Managing Complications of Foot and Ankle Surgery
Scott Ellis, *Editor*

MARCH 2022
Alternatives to Ankle Joint Replacement
Woo-Chun Lee, *Editor*

December 2021
Foot Ankle Deformity in the Child
Maurizio De Pellegrin, *Editor*

RELATED SERIES

Orthopedic Clinics
Clinics in Sports Medicine
Physical Medicine and Rehabilitation Clinics

THE CLINICS ARE NOW AVAILABLE ONLINE!
Access your subscription at:
www.theclinics.com

Foreword

Shooting Star: A Tribute to Alexej Barg

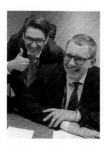

Cesar de Cesar Netto, MD, PhD
Consulting Editor

The last couple of months have been very hard for the Foot and Ankle Surgery Community, which was shocked by the unexpected news of Alexej Barg's passing. Our specialty lost one of its most prominent and brilliant names, with research contributions that have substantially changed our way of thinking, optimized the understanding of multiple pathologies, and improved the care of patients. *Foot and Ankle Clinics of North America* Editorial, unfortunately, lost its most passionate and excited Associate Editor. I have lost a great mentor and friend, and the void that he leaves in my heart will never be completely fulfilled.

Alexej attended medical School in Münster (Germany), Vienna (Austria), and Basel (Switzerland) and completed his residency and fellowship in renowned institutions in Switzerland and in the United States. He practiced as a Faculty at the University of Utah for several years, and in the last couple of years, he headed the Foot and Ankle Division at the University of Hamburg in Germany. Alexej was also the immediate past president of the International Weight-Bearing CT Society, where we interacted on a weekly/monthly basis for the last 4 to 5 years.

As previously mentioned, Alexej's contributions to the Foot and Ankle Specialty are impressive and unparallel for an extremely young investigator. With almost 260 publications, 5000 citations, and 330 coauthors, Alexej was like a shooting star or a comet that came, lit up our sky, marvelously marked his presence, and then left quicker than we all would like, like in a blink of an eye.

Alexej was just the nicest guy. A true gentleman. Incapable of saying negative things about anything or anyone. Always positive. Always available as a friend and as a colleague. An outstanding mentor and supporter of the young. An innovative mind. A hard worker. A genius.

He recently shared with me that one of his utmost passions was the *Foot and Ankle Clinics of North America* journal. He told me that the number one source of Foot and

Foot Ankle Clin N Am 27 (2022) xiii–xiv
https://doi.org/10.1016/j.fcl.2022.07.003
1083-7515/22/© 2022 Published by Elsevier Inc.

Ankle Surgery information he acquired throughout his training and career were the articles of *Foot and Ankle Clinics of North America*.

Alexej had a collection of all the journals' electronic articles as well as a large series of printed versions. When I started as the Consulting Editor for the journal, Alexej literally asked me to send him a signed version of the initial issue, with a dedicatory that he actually treasured in his office in Germany. I can't really recall seeing Alexej happier or more excited than when I invited him to serve as an Associate Editor for the journal. He was ecstatic and so passionate about it, incredibly supportive, and willing to do whatever was needed to continue the outstanding work of our journal. Now, without you, Alexej, we will do our best to continue to make you proud of our articles and contributions to Foot and Ankle science.

The memories will stay and last forever. His contributions will continue to echo for a long time.

Thank you, Alexej, so much for your kindness and friendship. Wherever you are, please continue to light up the environment with your blessed soul and powerful smile. We will miss you forever. I'll miss you forever, my great friend.

Our deepest condolences to Alexej's wife, parents, family, friends, colleagues, and admirers.

Cesar de Cesar Netto, MD, PhD
Orthopaedics and Rehabilitation
University of Iowa
Iowa City, IA, USA

E-mail address:
cesar-netto@uiowa.edu

Preface

Dear Foot and Ankle Surgeons!

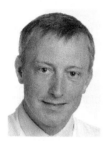

Fabian Krause, MD
Editor

Even though there is extended knowledge on how to prevent diabetes and its complications, how to control blood sugar levels, and how to treat diabetes-related complications in combination with a rising awareness that healthy nutrition is important to avoid diabetes mellitus, the prevalence of diabetes mellitus in our aging population is increasing all over the world. The prevalence of diabetes mellitus ranges from 13.3% in Mexico to 3.2% in Ireland, and in the United States, more than 30 million Americans, representing 12% of the population, has the condition.[1] Of these diabetics, 20% to 25% will develop diabetic foot ulcer as a frequent complication, mainly due to diabetic neuropathy, diabetic angiopathy, foot deformity–related abnormal plantar load distribution, and shear stress.[2]

Infection is a common complication of diabetic foot ulcers, with up to 58% of ulcers being infected at initial presentation at a diabetic foot clinic, rising to 82% in patients hospitalized for a diabetic foot ulcer.[3] These diabetic foot infections are associated with poor clinical outcomes for the patient and high costs for both patients and health care systems.[4] Patients with a diabetic foot infection have a 50-fold increased risk of hospitalization and 150-fold increased risk of lower-extremity amputation as opposed to patients with diabetes but no foot infection.[5] Among patients with a diabetic foot infection, about 5% will need a major amputation, and 20% to 30% will need a minor amputation, whereas the presence of peripheral arterial disease significantly increases amputation risk.[6]

Thus, chronic wounds and associated complications have major impacts for diabetic patients with regard to functional limitations, social participation, and quality of life. Direct and indirect health care costs for complication treatment, hospitalizations, amputations as well as rehabilitation or long-term disability represent a significant socioeconomic burden.

Since foot and ankle surgeons can't exert influence on this precarious evolution in the aging population, they need to do everything to improve patient education,

---

Foot Ankle Clin N Am 27 (2022) xv–xvi
https://doi.org/10.1016/j.fcl.2022.04.001
1083-7515/22/© 2022 Published by Elsevier Inc.

preemptive nonoperative and operative treatment of impending and existing diabetic foot complications, and secondary prophylaxis of recurrent complications. This *Foot and Ankle Clinics of North America* issue is dedicated to the diabetic foot and its complications. The issue contains new insights in improvements of diagnostics and nonoperative and operative treatment of diabetic foot complications of the last two decades and may assist the surgeon in advancing (interdisciplinary) nonoperative treatment options and increasing the success rates of surgery.

The world's most experienced foot and ankle surgeons dealing with the problems of the diabetic foot share their profound knowledge of the related nonoperative and operative treatment by contributing their articles to this *Foot and Ankle Clinics of North America* issue. So, please go ahead and enjoy the reading!

Fabian Krause, MD
Department of Orthopaedic Surgery
Inselspital, University of Berne
Freiburgstrasse
Berne, Switzerland

E-mail address:
fabian.krause@insel.ch

REFERENCES

1. Center for Disease Control and Prevention. National diabetes statistics report. Estimates of diabetes and its burden in the United States; 2017. Available at: https://www.cdc.gov/diabetes/data/statistics-report/.
2. Veves A, Murray HJ, Young MJ, et al. The risk of foot ulceration in diabetic patients with high foot pressure: a prospective study. Diabetologia 1992;35:660–3.
3. Prompers L, Huijberts M, Apelqvist J, et al. High prevalence of ischaemia, infection and serious comorbidity in patients with diabetic foot disease in Europe. Baseline results from the Eurodiale study. Diabetologia 2007;50:18–25.
4. Peters EJG, Lipsky BA. Diagnosis and management of infection in the diabetic foot. Med Clin North Am 2013;97:911–46.
5. Lavery LA, Armstrong DG, Wunderlich RP, et al. Risk factors for foot infections in individuals with diabetes. Diabetes Care 2006;29:1288–93.
6. Lipsky BA, Weigelt JA, Sun X, et al. Developing and validating a risk score for lower-extremity amputation in patients hospitalized for a diabetic foot infection. Diabetes Care 2011;34:1695–700.

Diagnostic Imaging of Diabetic Foot Disorders

Keivan Daneshvar, MD[a], Helen Anwander, MD[b],*

KEYWORDS

- Imaging • Radiography • MRI • CT

KEY POINTS

- In cellulitis, the presence of an abscess or osteomyelitis has to be searched.
- MRI is the gold standard diagnostic tool for osteomyelitis.
- It can be challenging to discriminate between osteomyelitis and bone marrow edema.

INTRODUCTION

Early and accurate diagnosis of diabetic foot pathologies, such as infection, neuro-arthropathy, and ischemia, is key in the successful treatment of patients with diabetic feet. Correct usage of various imaging modalities and knowledge of the different imaging findings are essential. Plain radiography, if possible, with full weight-bearing, is the preferred first-line imaging in the diabetic patient. Depending on the clinical suspicion, additional diagnostic imaging, such as computed tomography (CT), magnetic resonance imaging (MRI), and scintigraphy, is indicated. CT provides similar information as plain radiography, but with 3D reconstruction capabilities and with the possibility of contrast enhancement (CE). An iodinated contrast agent is used to enhance the visibility of internal structures as well as pathologies such as an abscess or angiopathy. Allergic reactions to the contrast agent are rare accounting for 0.6% of cases with only 0.04% considered severe.[1] The renal function has to be controlled before application of iodinated contrast agent as—particularly diabetic—patients with oftentimes impaired renal function are at risk for developing contrast-induced nephropathy.

Using MRI, the following 4 pulse sequences are the most often used: T1-weighted (T1w), T2-weighted (T2w), fluid sensitive sequences, for example, short-tau inversion recovery (STIR), and T1w with fat saturation (FS) and CE.

[a] Department of Diagnostic, Interventional and Pediatric Radiology, Inselspital, Bern University Hospital, University of Bern, Freiburgstrasse 18, 3010 Bern, Switzerland; [b] Department of Orthopaedic Surgery and Traumatology, Inselspital, Bern University Hospital, University of Bern, Freiburgstrasse 18, 3010 Bern, Switzerland
* Corresponding author.
E-mail address: helen.anwander@insel.ch

Foot Ankle Clin N Am 27 (2022) 513–527
https://doi.org/10.1016/j.fcl.2022.01.002
1083-7515/22/© 2022 The Author(s). Published by Elsevier Inc.

T2w imaging displays fluid as bright and fat as intermediate intense. In the STIR sequence, fluid is very bright; accordingly, it is useful to detect inflammation; however, the details are less well depicted on this sequence. T1w imaging displays anatomic features in detail. Fat (including bone marrow) is bright, liquid is dark. T1w imaging with fat suppression has a low signal in fatty and fluid areas and therefore is ideal for postcontrast imaging. Intravenous application of the contrast agent gadolinium will lead to hyperintensity in the area of hyperemia and inflammation. The nephrotoxicity of gadolinium is less than the contrast agent in CT scans, which is an advantage in diabetic patients, which often suffer from chronic renal failure.

Nuclear medicine techniques such as scintigraphy and, more recently, fluorine 18 fluorodeoxyglucose PET have demonstrated their ability to aid in bone marrow evaluation and provide functional information about the presence of osteomyelitis, when used alone or in combination with CT.[2,3] According to a recent meta-analysis, bone scanning has an 81% sensitivity in the detection of osteomyelitis in the diabetic foot but only a 28% specificity.[4] PET/MRI has been reported recently as a viable method for evaluating osteomyelitis in diabetic patients, and preliminary results are promising with a sensitivity of 100%.[5]

SOFT TISSUE PATHOLOGIES: CALLUS, ULCERATION, CELLULITIS, TISSUE ABSCESS

A diagnosis of callus and ulcer is mainly clinical. Plain radiography often does not display direct visualization of the ulcer, but sometimes a defect or swelling of the soft tissue. Callus and most ulcers evolve over an area with high pressure due to a bony prominence. Weight-bearing plain radiography of the foot is useful to locate these areas and find the underlying pathology leading to abnormal pressure distribution. Calcification of vessels may suggest underlying diabetic angiopathy. According to this, radiological imaging is not necessary for the diagnosis of callus or ulceration; however, it can be useful to find the underlying mechanic pathology for soft tissue pathologies and thereby the suitable operative or nonoperative therapy.

Swelling of the foot is a common finding in diabetic patients. There are many possible etiologies, including vascular insufficiency, peripheral neuropathy, and infection. Although cellulitis can be diagnosed clinically, further imaging is indicated if an underlying deep infection such as an abscess or osteomyelitis is suspected. The distinction between cellulitis, abscess, osteomyelitis, and Charcot arthropathy is clinically relevant, as in case of any deep infection, surgical treatment has to be evaluated. Standard radiography is not helpful in the diagnosis of an abscess.

Sonography is an ideal first-line imaging modality for the evaluation of cellulitis and soft tissue abscess. Healthy subcutaneous tissue is hypoechoic with few hyperechoic strands representing connective tissue. Increased thickness, increased echogenicity, and haziness of the subcutaneous tissue are signs of cellulitis. Progressive accumulation of edema in the connective tissue leads to striation and a "cobble-stone" appearance.[6] In ultrasound, fluid collections such as an abscess or a joint effusion can be demonstrated as anechoic or hypoechoic spherical findings with increased through-transmission. In case of an abscess, an echogenic capsule, as well as septa, may be seen. Furthermore, ultrasound can be used for the detection of foreign bodies, with a sensitivity higher than in MRI, especially if wooden.[7]

In the special case of necrotizing fasciitis, ultrasound can also be used to support the diagnosis. The findings are similar to cellulitis but more severe and with a thickened fascial layer and fluid tracking along the deep fascia. In addition, the finding of subcutaneous gas is pathognomonic for necrotizing fasciitis. The reliability of ultrasound in necrotizing fasciitis is high with sensitivity and specificity reaching 88%

and 93%, respectively.[8] However, the final diagnosis can only be made intraoperatively and no diagnostic procedure should delay the surgery.

In patients with cellulitis, CT can identify skin edema and subcutaneous fat stranding. Small collections may be found inside the diffusely affected soft tissue layers. An abscess typically shows a necrotic center and a well-defined fibrous capsule, which contains dilated blood vessels, and its postcontrast rim enhancement is pathognomonic.

The gold standard diagnostic modality for soft tissue pathologies is MRI. Callus appears as a focal prominence in the subcutaneous fat with low signal intensity in T1w and low to intermediate signal intensity on T2w sequences. Sometimes a bursa is formed below the callus, seen as fluid on MRI with low signal intensity in T1w and high intensity in T2w imaging. However, the bursa has no adjacent soft tissue reaction and no contrast agent enhancement and can thereby be distinguished from an abscess.[9] Ulcers appear as a soft tissue defect, bright on T2w sequences and with peripheral CE. A potential sinus tract to the bone has to be searched. After contrast administration, "tramtrack" enhancement of the sinus tract can be seen.

On MRI, soft tissue edema and cellulitis are seen as fat reticulation with intermediate signal intensity in T1w and high intensity in T2w images. In contrast to soft tissue edema, cellulitis is enhanced postcontrast. In a phlegmon, the subcutaneous fat shows ill-defined areas with low T1w and intermediate to high T2w and STIR signal intensity and vague post-CE. An abscess presents as a fluid collection area, often with rim enhancement after application of contrast agent. However, other findings such as a hematoma or a tumor can show a similar finding (**Table 1**).[10]

Areas of ischemia such as gangrene are seen in contrast-enhanced MRI as nonenhanced areas.

ADULT OSTEOMYELITIS

Plain radiographs are recommended as first-line imaging when osteomyelitis is suspected. Initial findings include soft tissue swelling and stranding of adjutant fat. The classic radiological triad including osteolysis, periosteal reaction, and bone destruction is generally not evident before a later stage at least 10 to 20 days after onset of symptoms.[11] Osteolysis is seen as small, ill-defined lucencies in the medullary bone and cortex (**Fig. 1**A). Cortical destruction may be evident. In a later stage, sequestration of dead, sclerotic bone can be found. In patients with implanted metal, sometimes a poorly marginated lucency can be found around the implant indicating hardware loosening. The shape of the lucency may help to discriminate between aseptic implant loosening and hardware-associated infection. While in case of infection, the bone lysis is round; in aseptic loosening, the lucency is conically shaped and starts at the point of most movement.[11] Sensitivity and specificity of plain radiography for osteomyelitis are 60% and 80%, respectively.[9] In serial radiographs, progressive change can support the diagnosis in uncertain cases. Gas might be seen in soft tissues, especially in cases with a sinus tract and adjacent osseous destruction (see **Fig 1**B).

If the clinical examination in combination with plain radiographs does not lead to a conclusion, MRI is the gold standard in patients with suspected osteomyelitis. Osteomyelitis is bright on STIR and T2w and confluent hypointense in T1w images. In contrast, bone marrow edema is also bright on T2w images but the T1w image has an intermediate to decreased reticulated hazy intensity (**Figs. 2** and **3**). Bone marrow enhancement after the administration of contrast agent is in favor of osteomyelitis.[12] Osteomyelitis in patients with diabetic foot syndrome is often in proximity to the entry point, such as an ulcer. However, bone marrow edema without osteomyelitis can also

Table 1
Key points of diagnostic imaging of diabetic foot disorders

Pathology	Radiography	CT	MRI	Sonography	Overall
Cellulitis	Soft tissue swelling, adjacent fat stranding, rarely soft tissue gas	Soft tissue swelling, adjacent fat obliteration and stranding, fluid collection, rarely soft tissue gas	T1w: low to intermediate SI T2w: high SI T1w with CE: thick rim enhancement	Increased echogenicity and haziness of subcutaneous tissue, possible fluid collection	Search for an abscess and adjacent osteomyelitis. Exclude tumor.
Acute osteomyelitis	Early: cortex indistinctness Advanced: osseous destruction, dense periosteal reaction Late: sequester and Brodie abscess	Osteolytic destruction, reactive bone formation, +/– soft tissue abscess Late: sequester and Brodie abscess	T1w: confluent low SI T2w + STIR: high SI CE: within bone and around abscess. +/– soft tissue abscess or gas	Not useful	Difficult differentiating between osteomyelitis and Charcot foot. Bone destruction faster in osteomyelitis than in tumor.
Bone marrow edema	Bone density is normal, unless decreased by diabetic or elderly patients.	Not useful	T1w: hazy low SI T2w + STIR: high SI CE: +/– thin rim in Charcot foot.	Not useful	Charcot foot might have fluid collections with enhancing rim in absence of osteomyelitis.
Septic arthritis	Early: normal Advanced: joint effusion and narrowing, periarticular osteoporosis, marginal erosions, sclerotic reaction.	Not modality of choice. Soft tissue swelling, joint effusion, articular narrowing, bone and cartilage erosions.	T1w: low SI T2w + STIR: high SI CE: subchondral adjacent to joint, thickened synovium, joint effusion, articular narrowing.	Highly sensitive for joint effusion, but not specific for septic effusion. Can guide aspiration.	With clinical suspicion, aspiration required. MRI examination must include postcontrast sequences.

Abbreviations: CE, contrast enhancement; CT, computed tomography; SI, signal intensity; T1w, T1 weighted; T2w, T2 weighted.

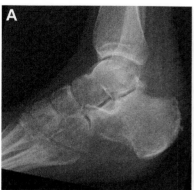
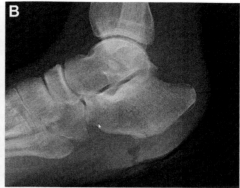

Fig. 1. (*A*) Lateral radiograph of the midfoot and hindfoot of a diabetic patient showing osteopenic changes. (*B*) Lateral radiograph of the midfoot and hindfoot (different patient than *A*) after partial resection of the calcaneus shows soft tissue swelling and gas inclusion in the soft tissue suggestive of pressure ulcer in the diabetic foot. The soft tissue defect dorsal of the calcaneus is suggestive of pressure ulcer. Dorsal of the ankle and around the plantar fascia, cortical lytic lesions due to osteomyelitis, and soft tissue swelling due to inflammation can be seen.

be found as a reaction to a soft tissue infection or an ulcer. Other signs of osteomyelitis include cortical interruption and enhancement at the margins of the periosteum indicating a periostitis. The sensitivity of MRI for osteomyelitis ranges between 77% and 100%, and specificity between 79% and 100%.[13,14] The application of gadolinium increases the accuracy of osteomyelitis from 78% to 89%.[15]

CT is not recommended as first-line modality to evaluate osteomyelitis; however, it can be helpful to evaluate other pathologies leading to soft tissue swelling in the foot, such as neuroarthropathy or an abscess. In late-stage osteomyelitis, periostitis,

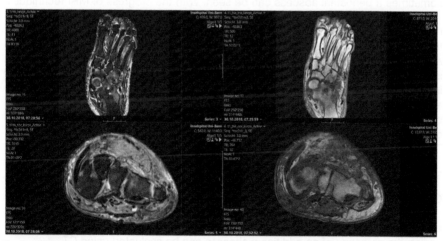

Fig. 2. MRI of a Charcot foot. (*A*) Upper left: long axis turbo inversion recovery magnitude (TIRM); (*B*) upper right T1 TSE long axis; (*C*) lower left: TIRM coronal short axis; and (*D*) lower right: T1 TSE short axis. Hyperintensities in TIRM and not confluent, stranding hypointensities in T1w in the midfoot are more suggestive of osseous reaction to Charcot joints than to an infection.

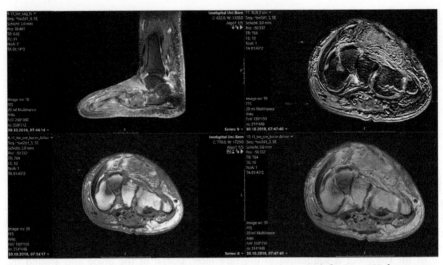

Fig. 3. The same patient in **Fig. 3** with a Charcot foot. (*A*) Upper left: T1w TSE fat suppression with CE; (*B*) upper right: CE subtraction short axis; (*C*) lower left: T1w TSE without CE coronal short axis; and (*D*) lower right: T1w TSE with CE coronal short axis. The diffuse hypointensities in the subcutis in T1w with CE in subtraction series and the slight post-CE of the midfoot and metatarsals are suggestive of inflammation and cellulitis around Charcot joints.

rarefication of bone or bone destruction can evolve and be seen on the CT scan. In chronic osteomyelitis, bony sequestrum can form, representing a central area with necrotic bone and granulation tissue around it. On CT, sequestra are seen as a dense bone spicule in the medullary cavity surrounded by soft tissue density.[16] If MRI is available, ultrasound is not recommended as a diagnostic tool for osteomyelitis. However, sometimes a periosteal abscess can be seen. With the progress of MRI techniques, the role of scintigraphy in the diagnosis of osteomyelitis is limited. Technetium (99mTc) 3-phase bone scan can differentiate between cellulitis and osteomyelitis.[11] In cellulitis, tracer activity increases in the early images but is normal in delayed images, 2 to 4 hours after application. Noninflammatory bone conditions such as ischemic necrosis demonstrate normal activity in early images and increased activity in delayed images. Osteomyelitis results in high activity in both, early and delayed images. It has to be kept in mind that the diabetic foot can have vascular problems; decreased blood flow will lead to false-negative results and, on the other hand, pathologies with hyperemia will lead to false-positive results.

SEPTIC ARTHRITIS

One-third of patients with pedal osteomyelitis have adjacent septic arthritis.

On plain radiography as well as on a CT scan, septic arthritis may be seen as joint effusion, articular narrowing, and, in a chronic stage, joint destruction. As discussed earlier, the presence of an additional abscess can be evaluated using CT.

On MRI, the findings are similar with also joint effusion and articular narrowing due to cartilage destruction. Furthermore, the synovia is usually thickened with intense CE. Sometimes a sinus tract can be found. Periarticular osteopenia due to hyperemia and direct communication of joint fluid with an adjacent sinus tract may be present. The

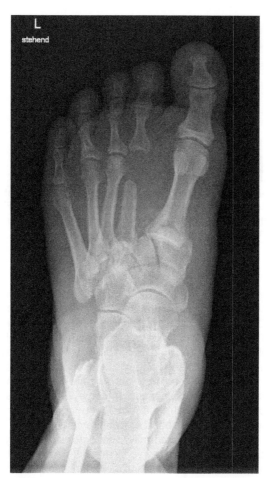

Fig. 4. AP radiograph in a diabetic Charcot foot with prior amputation of the distal meta-tarsal II. 5Ds findings on the midfoot: normal bone density, joint distension, bony debris, joint disorganization, and dislocation

adjacent soft tissues may show perisynovial edema, in addition to subchondral marrow with a thin rim of reactive marrow edema and marginal erosions. The difference between reactive edema and osteomyelitis has to be evaluated carefully. As described earlier, both are bright in STIR and T2w images, but while osteomyelitis is confluent and intense T1w hypointense, bone marrow edema shows an intermediate, hazy and reticulated intensity in T1w images; however, there is significant overlap. Furthermore, a proximal extension beyond the subchondral bone also is a sign of osteomyelitis. Joint aspiration is required to confirm the diagnosis.

CHARCOT ARTHROPATHY

Charcot arthropathy refers to a progressive and destructive disorder affecting the joints, bones, and soft tissue in diabetic feet. The pathology is discussed in detail in the according article. In imaging, the diagnosis of Charcot arthropathy includes 5Ds: bone density, bony debris, joint distension, joint disorganization, and dislocation

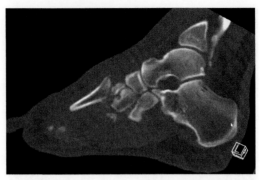

Fig. 5. Sagittal reconstruction of noncontrast enhancement CT in a diabetic Charcot foot with prior amputation of the distal metatarsal II, the same patient as **Fig. 4**. 5Ds findings on the midfoot: normal bone density, joint distension, bony debris, joint disorganization, and dislocation, there is diffuse swelling of soft tissue around midfoot.

(**Figs. 4** and **5**). The prevalence of this arthropathy is not distributed equally in all joints but is found in the following order: Lisfranc joint > talonavicular joint > Chopart joint > intercuneiform and naviculocuneiform joints. Conventional radiographs are important for staging and monitoring Charcot arthropathy. Eichenholtz classification[17] is a historical, widely used system based on radiological findings. In stage 1, the developmental stage, the following findings appear: focal bone demineralization and fragmentation of subchondral bone, leading to periarticular debris formation or fractures and finally joint subluxation and dislocation. In stage 2, the coalescence stage, the debris is absorbed, new periosteal bone forms, and large fragments fuse. Stage 3, the remodeling stage, displays the final stage with remodeled bone, new bone formation, and possibly gross residual deformity. Standard radiography is important for monitoring progression, but it cannot serve to rule out Charcot arthropathy. Shibata and colleagues[18] proposed a stage 0, the inflammation stage, before stage 1 according to Eichenholtz. In stage 0, clinical signs such as erythema and changes in MRI are present but there are no changes in standard radiography evident yet. Correct diagnosis and treatment in this stage are critical to prevent further progression and final foot deformity.[19] Stage 0 on MRI is seen as subchondral edema with or without microfracture, leading to intraarticular debris and subchondral cysts. Also, soft tissue edema, fluid collections, and effusion may be present. Bone marrow will show post-CE. The bone marrow edema appears as hypointensity to intermediate hazy intensity in T1w images and hyperintensity in T2w and STIR images. This mimics the changes seen in osteomyelitis, the most important differential diagnosis to Charcot arthropathy. Findings, which help to distinguish between the 2 diagnoses are the following: Charcot arthropathy favors the midfoot and is often periarticular in multiple joints involved, whereas osteomyelitis is characterized by focal involvement of weight-bearing surfaces including the toes, metatarsal heads, and calcaneus and is often in proximity to an ulcer. Charcot arthropathy leads to cysts and fragmentation; osteomyelitis is associated with cortical lesions. T1w images in osteomyelitis show confluent and prominent hypointensity. CT scan is not the first choice for the diagnosis of Charcot arthropathy, but it can be used to show bone changes including fragmentation, bone remodeling new bone formation in more detail than plain radiographs. Subsequently, it is useful for preoperative planning.

MUSCLE DISORDERS IN DIABETIC FEET

Diabetic individuals can develop a variety of muscular problems, including diabetic muscle ischemia (DMI), viral and inflammatory myositis, and muscle denervation. Although muscle edema is a frequent imaging finding in all of these disorders, the clinical symptoms, anatomic distribution, and imaging findings associated with each vary.

Diabetic Muscle Infarction

DMI, also known as diabetic myonecrosis or diabetic muscle infarction, is a type of end-organ complication that arises in people with long-term, poorly managed diabetes and is associated with nephropathy and neuropathy.[20] The clinical onset of DMI is abrupt, with significant thigh or calf pain and swelling that develops over days or weeks,[21] however, in absence of leukocytosis or fever. A palpable lump can also be present. The cause of DMI is unknown, but microangiopathy has been suggested as a possible cause.[22] Muscle fiber necrosis and edema are evident on pathologic examination, along with fibrinous blockage of arterioles and capillaries. The preferred modality for evaluating patients suspected of having DMI is MRI. In acute and subacute phases: in STIR and T2w hyperintensity with fascicular enlargement. Muscle enhancement is common, with hypoenhancement or nonenhancement in the core regions. In chronic phase: atrophic-appearing fascicles with intraepineurial fatty changes. Muscle infarction shows hyperintense muscle swelling on MR with adjacent soft tissue reaction. The thigh is the most common location for myopathy ($\geq$80%); the calf is the second most common site. The symptoms might be unilateral or bilateral, and they usually manifest themselves in noncontiguous muscles in the thighs and calves.[21]

Infectious and Inflammatory Myositis

Diabetic patients are susceptible to infectious pyomyositis, a disease caused by the hematogenous spread of bacteria to muscle, due to underlying immunologic failure.[23] When DMI is suspected in a patient, this entity is an important differential diagnostic consideration. Although the imaging appearances of the 2 entities may be similar, the presence of smooth-walled intramuscular abscesses with rim-like enhancement favors the diagnosis of pyomyositis over DMI. Areas of muscular ischemia or necrosis, on the other hand, tend to appear heterogeneous in DMI, with linear enhancement streaks crossing central nonenhancing areas surrounded by widespread regions of enhancing muscle.[24] Fever, leukocytosis with a left shift, increased inflammatory markers, and bacteremia are clinical characteristics that favor the diagnosis of infectious pyomyositis over DMI. It is necessary to distinguish between DMI and pyomyositis because the latter requires antibiotics and abscess drainage. Findings of bilateral symmetric edema in the proximal muscles, especially those in the pelvis and thighs, on MRI can assist diagnose inflammatory myopathy and determine its severity.[25] Muscle biopsy based solely on clinical markers has a 25% false-negative rate. By making it easier to select damaged muscles for sampling, MRI improves diagnostic yield. Inflammatory myositis is frequently accompanied by skin lesions. Clinical history, physical examination, muscle enzyme tests, and muscle biopsy with immunostaining are used to make the diagnosis.

Muscle Denervation

Muscle denervation has a variety of causes, one of the most frequent is due to diabetic peripheral neuropathy. T2w images show signal hyperintensity in the afflicted muscles and is a marker of subacute muscular denervation, although T1w images show normal signal intensity and architecture.[26] Muscles with chronic denervation exhibit decreased mass and fatty infiltration, which is best seen on T1w imaging. In diabetic patients, subacute or chronic denervation appears early and conspicuously, usually affecting the foot's intrinsic musculature. Denervation induced by diabetic peripheral neuropathy can be distinguished from that caused by DMI by the presence of muscles within a peripheral nerve distribution, the absence of concomitant fascial edema, and the presence of peripheral neuropathy at physical examination.

CALCANEUS INSUFFICIENCY FRACTURE

A neuropathic avulsion fracture of the tuberosity in a patient with long-term diabetes mellitus is significant sequelae.[27] The fracture occurs in these patients without a history of major trauma or overuse activity. The primary fracture line runs parallel to the apophyseal scar, and the fracture usually affects the superior cortex, although not always. In addition, the fracture tends to spread posteriorly, with a horizontal component directly distal to the Achilles tendon insertion..[28] Distraction and fragmentation are common findings when imaging the fracture sequentially. Neuropathic fractures are important because they have a much higher rate of infection, nonunion, malunion, and fixation failure than nonneuropathic insufficiency fractures, and they take much longer to heal. The MRI shows low signal fracture line with displacement of posterior tuberosity fragment in T1w images and on fluid-sensitive sequences, for example, TIRM, a high signal fracture line with surrounding bone edema.

TARSAL/METATARSAL STRESS FRACTURE

Foot overuse injuries are an issue in diabetic patients with inadequate pain sensitivity due to diabetic polyneuropathy; accordingly, they may not notice the overuse. An early stress injury may proceed to a complete fracture if the mechanical load is maintained

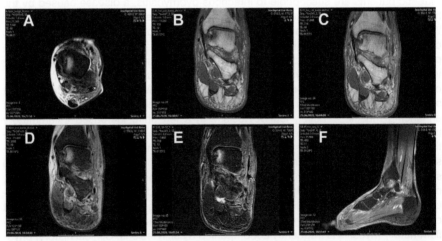

Fig. 6. MRI of diabetic foot with pressure ulcer. (A) Upper left: axial STIR; hyperintensity on medial talus indicates edema. (B) Upper middle: T1w TSE coronal without contrast-enhanced (CE); shows confluent T1w hypointensity, suggestive of osteomyelitis. (C) Upper right: T1w TSE coronal with CE; shows CE in medial of talus, in addition, there is soft tissue swelling with CE on lateral of ankle. (D) Lower left: coronal STIR; hyperintensity on medial talus indicates edema. (E) Lower middle: subtraction coronal with CE; shows CE in medial of talus, in addition, there is soft tissue swelling with CE on lateral of ankle including soft tissue defect on pressure ulcer. (F) Lower right: T1 TSE FS sagittal with CE. CE in medial of talus.

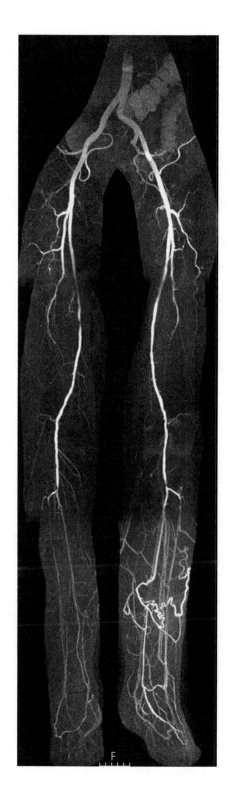

and there is no protective sensation. Early detection and treatment of stress fractures, such as unloading and immobilization, can reduce the risk of development to stage 1 Charcot arthropathy, which causes bone breakdown or complete fracture, as well as irreversible foot deformities and amputation. The most common imaging modality for identifying stress fractures is radiography; however, early bone stress injuries may not be visible. The most sensitive method for identifying stress injuries is MRI. MRI is particularly sensitive in detecting bone bruising, bone marrow edema, and microfractures associated with chronic stress responses. MRI offers useful information about the surrounding soft tissues, too. Bone marrow edema is a nonspecific characteristic that can occur in osteomyelitis, tumors, and bone bruises and is an early marker of stress-related bone damage. In individuals with neuropathy, foot edema should be checked and stress fracture should be considered as differential diagnosis.

AMYLOID AND CRYSTAL DEPOSITION

In diabetic, end-stage renal disease patients, renal osteodystrophy secondary to diabetes mellitus is common. Renal osteodystrophy may show altered bone density, resorptive patterns on all bone, mainly in hands, cranium, and distal clavicles. They show nodular soft tissue densities. Periarticular amyloid, sodium urate, and hydroxyapatite depositions are common in patients on dialysis.

REVIEWING THE IMAGING MODALITIES
Radiography

Plain, full weight-bearing radiography is the preferred first-line imaging in the diabetic patient to assess the alignment of the foot, bony prominences as cause of ulcers, and potential fractures and joint dislocations. It is widely acknowledged that radiography is insensitive to the early stages of osteomyelitis.[1,2] Bone infection can occur up to 4 weeks before radiological changes, though most changes occur within a couple of weeks. Serial radiographs can be very convincing if they show progressive bone resorption, cortical destruction, and periosteal elevation. There have been no formal evaluations of the role of serial radiographs in the diagnosis of osteomyelitis that we are aware of. Furthermore, other clinical conditions common in diabetic patients, such as gout and Charcot osteoarthropathy, may complicate radiographic interpretation.

CT Scan

Although CT has a limited function in the imaging of diabetes-related foot problems, it does have some advantages over radiography, such as the ability to provide pictures with high tissue contrast. Furthermore, it is more sensitive and specific for detecting cortical erosions, tiny sequestra, soft tissue gas, calcifications, and foreign bodies when compared with radiography. The presence of ionizing radiation, as well as insufficient differentiation of healthy and sick tissues, are the fundamental limitations of CT.

Fig. 7. MR angiography in a patient with chronic pressure ulcer along with calcaneal osteomyelitis due to diabetic foot syndrome with peripheral artery disease on the right lower leg and concomitant chronic venous insufficiency on the left lower leg.

MRI

MRI is currently recognized as an effective modality for assessing soft tissue and bone marrow changes associated with diabetic foot.[12,13] MRI has a high sensitivity and specificity (90%–100% and 40%–100%, respectively) for detecting bone marrow edema as an early finding of neuroarthropathy[14] (**Fig 6**). The main advantages of MRI for detecting and delineating the extent of an infection are its high soft tissue contrast and multiplanar imaging capabilities. MRI can also help to distinguish osteomyelitis from neuroarthropathy and reactive bone marrow edema, as well as sterile joint effusion from septic arthritis, all of which require entirely different treatment.

Angiography

Peripheral arterial disease is common in patients with diabetic foot syndrome with a prevalence of 50% in patients with foot ulcers. It is a known risk factor for inferior outcome.[29,30] Subsequently, the adequate diagnosis and therapy if necessary are important for optimal patient care. Angiography is indicated in patients with diabetic foot syndrome in the case of suspected or known peripheral arterial disease, with non-healing ulcers and preoperative for optimization of the postoperative wound healing.

Conventional peripheral angiography is performed by injection of an iodinated contrast agent over the femoral artery, followed by fluoroscopic assessment of the distribution of the contrast agent in the arteries. A stenosis can be diagnosed and treated accordingly. MR angiography is also helpful in diagnosis and follow-up of the patients (**Fig 7**).

Nuclear Medicine

In early phase of osteomyelitis, the sensitivity of a 3 (or 4) phase bisphosphonate-linked technetium bone scan is greater than that of radiography. However, specificity[1,6,7] (averaging 50%) is poor because almost any type of bone disorder (including neuroarthropathy and healing osteomyelitis) can cause increased isotope uptake on a bone scan. As a result, some authorities have concluded that positive technetium bone scans do not significantly increase the likelihood of disease, while negative ones do not significantly decrease it, and that this modality should be used sparingly.[8] Other radionuclide imaging agents, such as scans using white blood cells (labeled autologous leukocytes), labeled immunoglobulin, or other infection-specific radio pharmaceuticals, are more specific than technetium bone scans.[9,10] They can help differentiate osteomyelitis from soft tissue infection or Charcot-type changes but their sensitivity is limited.[11] They lack spatial resolution, are expensive, and technically demanding, and should be regarded as special-purpose problem-solving tools rather than first- or second-line modalities.

CLINICS CARE POINTS

- Start with weight-bearing radiography of the foot.
- In case of a soft tissue infection such as cellulitis, search for an abscess.
- If the clinical examination in combination with plain radiography does not lead to a conclusion regarding possible osteomyelitis, the next imaging modality recommended is MRI if available.
- To differentiate between osteomyelitis and aseptic bone marrow edema, assess T1w images on MRI: osteomyelitis will appear as confluent low signal intensity, bone marrow edema as

reticulated, hazy low to intermediate signal intensity.

DISCLOSURE

The authors have nothing to disclose.

REFERENCES

1. Wang CL, Cohan RH, Ellis JH, et al. Frequency, outcome, and appropriateness of treatment of nonionic iodinated contrast media reactions. AJR Am J Roentgenol 2008;191(2):409–15.
2. Palestro CJ, Mehta HH, Patel M, et al. Marrow versus infection in the Charcot joint: indium-111 leukocyte and technetium-99m sulfur colloid scintigraphy. J Nucl Med 1998;39(2):346–50.
3. Höpfner S, Krolak C, Kessler S, et al. Preoperative imaging of Charcot neuroarthropathy in diabetic patients: comparison of ring PET, hybrid PET, and magnetic resonance imaging. Foot Ankle Int 2004;25(12):890–5.
4. Khodaee M, Lombardo D, Montgomery LC, et al. Clinical inquiry: what's the best test for underlying osteomyelitis in patients with diabetic foot ulcers? J Fam Pract 2015;64(5):309–10, 321.
5. Yaddanapudi K, Matthews R, Brunetti V, et al. PET-MRI in diagnosing pedal osteomyelitis in diabetic patients. J Nucl Med 2015;56(suppl 3):307.
6. Adhikari S, Blaivas M. Sonography first for subcutaneous abscess and cellulitis evaluation. J Ultrasound Med 2012;31(10):1509–12.
7. Horton LK, Jacobson JA, Powell A, et al. Sonography and radiography of soft-tissue foreign bodies. AJR Am J Roentgenol 2001;176(5):1155–9.
8. Yen ZS, Wang HP, Ma HM, et al. Ultrasonographic screening of clinically-suspected necrotizing fasciitis. Acad Emerg Med 2002;9(12):1448–51.
9. Donovan A, Schweitzer ME. Current concepts in imaging diabetic pedal osteomyelitis. Radiol Clin North Am 2008;46(6):1105–24, vii.
10. Morrison WB, Schweitzer ME, Batte WG, et al. Osteomyelitis of the foot: relative importance of primary and secondary MR imaging signs. Radiology 1998;207(3):625–32.
11. Crim JR, Seeger LL. Imaging evaluation of osteomyelitis. Crit Rev Diagn Imaging 1994;35(3):201–56.
12. Donovan A, Schweitzer ME. Use of MR imaging in diagnosing diabetes-related pedal osteomyelitis. Radiographics 2010;30(3):723–36.
13. Tsang KW, Morrison WB. Update: Imaging of Lower Extremity Infection. Semin Musculoskelet Radiol 2016;20(2):175–91.
14. Kapoor A, Page S, Lavalley M, et al. Magnetic resonance imaging for diagnosing foot osteomyelitis: a meta-analysis. Arch Intern Med 2007;167(2):125–32.
15. Morrison WB, Schweitzer ME, Wapner KL, et al. Osteomyelitis in feet of diabetics: clinical accuracy, surgical utility, and cost-effectiveness of MR imaging. Radiology 1995;196(2):557–64.
16. Gold RH, Tong DJ, Crim JR, et al. Imaging the diabetic foot. Skeletal Radiol 1995;24(8):563–71.
17. Eichenholtz SN. Charcot joints. Springfield, IL, USA: Charles C. Thomas; 1966.
18. Shibata T, Tada K, Hashizume C. The results of arthrodesis of the ankle for leprotic neuroarthropathy. J Bone Joint Surg Am 1990;72(5):749–56.

19. Wukich DK, Sung W. Charcot arthropathy of the foot and ankle: modern concepts and management review. J Diabetes Complications 2009;23(6):409–26.
20. Umpierrez GE, Stiles RG, Kleinbart J, et al. Diabetic muscle infarction. Am J Med 1996;101(3):245–50.
21. Jelinek JS, Murphey MD, Aboulafia AJ, et al. Muscle infarction in patients with diabetes mellitus: MR imaging findings. Radiology 1999;211(1):241–7.
22. Trujillo-Santos AJ. Diabetic muscle infarction: an underdiagnosed complication of long-standing diabetes. Diabetes Care 2003;26(1):211–5.
23. Belsky DS, Teates CD, Hartman ML. Case report: diabetes mellitus as a predisposing factor in the development of pyomyositis. Am J Med Sci 1994;308(4):251–4.
24. Kattapuram TM, Suri R, Rosol MS, et al. Idiopathic and diabetic skeletal muscle necrosis: evaluation by magnetic resonance imaging. Skeletal Radiol 2005;34(4):203–9.
25. May DA, Disler DG, Jones EA, et al. Abnormal signal intensity in skeletal muscle at MR imaging: patterns, pearls, and pitfalls. RadioGraphics 2000;20(Spec Issue):S295–315.
26. Kamath S, Venkatanarasimha N, Walsh MA, et al. MRI appearance of muscle denervation. Skeletal Radiol 2008;37(5):397–404.
27. El-Khoury GY, Kathol MH. Neuropathic fractures in patients with diabetes mellitus. Radiology 1980;134:313–6.
28. Kathol MH, El-Khoury GY, Moore TE, et al. Calcaneal insufficiency avulsion fractures in patients with diabetes mellitus. Radiology 1991;180:725–9.
29. Prompers L, Huijberts M, Apelqvist J, et al. High prevalence of ischaemia, infection and serious comorbidity in patients with diabetic foot disease in Europe. Baseline results from the Eurodiale study. Diabetologia 2007;50(1):18–25.
30. Armstrong DG, Lavery LA, Harkless LB. Validation of a diabetic wound classification system. The contribution of depth, infection, and ischemia to risk of amputation. Diabetes Care 1998;21(5):855–9.

The Interdisciplinary Approach
Preventive and Therapeutic Strategies for Diabetic Foot Ulcers

Christophe Kurze, MD[a,*], Chui Jia Farn, MD[a,b], James Siow, MD[a,c]

KEYWORDS

- Interdisciplinary management • Diabetic foot ulceration • Prevention • Therapy
- Diabetes mellitus

KEY POINTS

- Coordinated care between different levels of care is key in the management of diabetic foot ulcer (DFU) patients.
- An interdisciplinary team approach optimises the evaluation and treatment process of DFU patients and has been shown to improve outcomes such as amputation rates, length of hospital stay and mortality rates.
- Early identification and management of risk factors can improve healing and reduce recurrence of DFUs.
- Treatment requires a targeted approach involving an interdisciplinary team of experts of doctors, nurses and allied health professionals.
- Prevention of DFU involves patients and their relatives and strategies should be instituted at all levels of care and continued in the primary care.

PREVALENCE OF DIABETIC FOOT ULCERS AND HEALTH CARE COSTS

The average global prevalence of diabetic foot ulcers (DFUs) is 6.3% with an increasing trend. The lifetime risk of a diabetic developing a DFU is between 19% and 34% based on a study by Armstrong and colleagues.[1] There are also considerable regional differences in the world, with North America having the highest prevalence of DFUs at 13%, Africa at 7.2%, Asia and Europe at 5.5% and 5.1%, respectively, and Oceania with the lowest at 3.0%.[2] Within 5 years of the first occurrence of a DFU, 50% to

The authors have nothing to disclose.
[a] Department of Orthopedic Surgery, Inselspital, University of Berne, Freiburgstrasse, 3010 Berne, Switzerland; [b] Department of Orthopedic Surgery, National Taiwan University Hospital, Taipei, Taiwan; [c] Department of Orthopedic Surgery, Woodlands Health, Singapore
* Corresponding author.
E-mail address: Christophe.kurze@insel.ch

Foot Ankle Clin N Am 27 (2022) 529–543
https://doi.org/10.1016/j.fcl.2022.03.001
1083-7515/22/© 2022 The Authors. Published by Elsevier Inc. This is an open access article under the CC BY-NC-ND license (http://creativecommons.org/licenses/by-nc-nd/4.0/).

70% of patients in the United States will die and 5% will require a major amputation.[3] Worldwide, it is estimated that DFUs occur every 1.2 seconds, and amputations are performed every 30 seconds.[4] As a result, there is a significant economic burden, with treatment and follow-up costs of DFUs (not including the treatment of diabetes mellitus per se) in North America estimated at $ 9 to 13 billion annually.[5,6]

INTERDISCIPLINARY DIABETIC FOOT CLINIC
Tasks of an Interdisciplinary Team

The main tasks of an interdisciplinary diabetic foot clinic (IDFC) are the treatment of existing DFUs, secondary prevention, prevention of recurrences, and sometimes primary preventions.

The percentage of patients with DFU with peripheral artery disease (PAD) ranges from close to 50% to more than 50% based on current literature.[7,8] Hence, early and appropriate diagnostic evaluation of the extent and localization of the peripheral vascular disease should be done. Early vascular interventions should also be performed if indicated after assessing for contraindications. In noninfected ulcers, which are usually superficial, local surgical debridement, diabetic wound care under a specialist nurse or podiatrist, and appropriate footwear including an off-loading orthosis are prescribed as early as possible. In infected ulcers, which are usually deep, early and aggressive wound debridement is necessary for infection source control and to prevent proximal and systemic progression of infection. For such patients, the IDFC should arrange for hospitalization and start broad-spectrum intravenous antibiotics early. During surgery, numerous deep tissue biopsies allow the team and especially the ID specialist to identify the pathogen, check for bacterial resistance, and to administer the most appropriate antibiotics. The ID specialist's expertise will be crucial when there is the presence of multidrug-resistant bacteria or when patients have contraindications to culture-specific antibiotics. Therefore, the IDFC's access to such expertise should be readily available.[9]

For patients with a high risk of recurrent DFUs, it is key for the endocrinologist to optimize glycemic control and titrate diabetic medications. Next, intensive patient education by a diabetes educator is also vital in reducing the likelihood of recurrence.[10] Further preventive strategies include footwear advice or modification, orthotics, and podiatry care for calluses.

The management of complications of diabetes mellitus such as retinopathy or nephropathy, although not the primary task of the IDFC, should be actively recognized and referred to the respective disciplines for further management.

Optimal Composition of an Interdisciplinary Diabetic Foot Clinic

It has been shown that having an interdisciplinary foot care team along with evidence-based prevention and management reduces the frequency of diabetes-related lower extremity amputation. However, based on a systematic review by Musuuza and colleagues,[3] there is a large variability in the composition of these teams worldwide. The investigators evaluated the optimal composition of an interdisciplinary team and concluded that teams with members who can optimize glycemic control, manage foot wounds, vascular disease, and wound infection are associated with a reduced risk of major amputation, although further studies are still required to clarify the core members.

Graded Team Size

The International Working Group on the Diabetic Foot (IWGDF) guidelines[11] recommend a breakdown into 3 levels of teams (**Table 1**). The first level is a local basic

Table 1	
Graded team size according to the International Working Group on the Diabetic Foot guidelines	
Level of Care	**Specialists Involved**
Level 1	General practitioner, podiatrist, diabetic nurse
Level 2	Level 1 and surgeon (foot and ankle, general), endocrinologist, vascular specialist (angiologist und vascular surgeon), infectious dieases specialist, shoe and orthotic technician
Level 3	Level 2 working together in an interdisciplinary way with special expertise in diabetic patients

Data from Schaper et al.[11]

care team, which should be widely available and accessible. A regional team forms the second level, and a tertiary center with a specialized interdisciplinary care setup forms the third level team. The number and expertise of team members involved increases with every level. The first level should be incorporated within the local primary medical care team. The team should consist of podiatrists, wound experts/diabetes nurses, and general practitioners to carry out regular checkups and administer basic routine treatment.[11] Complicated cases or those with a poor outcome should be referred to the next higher level of care. Ultimately, successfully treated cases at centers with level 2 and 3 teams are referred back to the local basic team (level 1) to allow for equitable patient distribution. In a level 2 team, the endocrinologist is probably the most important team member as early treatment and intensive control of diabetes mellitus is one of the major factors in the treatment of DFUs[12,13] and to prevent secondary diabetic complications. Surgical disciplines such as orthopedic, general, and vascular surgeons should ideally be on site. If necessary, interdisciplinary diabetes specialists and podiatrists, as well as shoe technicians and orthotists, should be available. The main difference between a level 2 and level 3 team is that the specialists are on-site at the same time, work together in a coordinated way, and specialize in treating patients with DFU. Ideally, an IDFC and inpatient interdisciplinaryrounds including specialists of level 1 to 3 teams are established in level 3 centers.[14]

Advantages of the Interdisciplinary Team

Interdisciplinary teamwork optimizes efficiency and expedites the evaluation and treatment of patients. In addition, these specialists deal with complex problems on a routine basis with regular communication that helps to accelerate decision-making processes. Clinic-specific algorithms or pathways help to streamline and coordinate the different tasks within the IDFC and help to optimize each patient visit. Furthermore, important diagnostics such as radiographs or vascular workups are carried out in a timely and coordinated manner. The organization of the IDFC depends on the individual hospital's requirements, workflow, and infrastructure. Thus, these processes differ greatly among various clinics worldwide, and there cannot be general recommendations for a consistent organization process.[3,14]

Objectively, with the implementation of an IDFC, 94% of the centers reduced their rate of amputations.[3] Furthermore, length of hospital stay and mortality rates were also reduced with the implementation of IDFCs[15]; this would in turn reduce the

Table 2
Types of ulcer and clinical manifestation

	Neurogenic Ulcer	Venous Ulcer	Arterial Ulcer
Appearance limb	Sensory dysfunction foot deformity	Edema, hyperpigmentation, varicose, eczematous dermatitis	Pale and dry skin, prolonged capillary reperfusion
Location	Pressure exposed region	Malleolar region, tibia	Pressure exposed region, tiptoe
Characteristics	Deep ulcer with reddish base and easy bleeding	Wide range, less necrotic tissue, exudate	Deep ulcer, necrosis, pale ground
Pulse	Mostly normal pulse	Normal pulse and skin temperature	Weak or absent pulse, pale skin
Pain	No relevant pain	Mild or moderate pain that elevated leg	Moderate to strong pain that improves with rest or lowering the leg

Data from Wang et al.[14]

economic burden of the disease. Consequently, various national and international guidelines emphasize the advantages of interdisciplinary teamwork in the treatment of patients with DFU.

DIAGNOSTICS OF DIABETIC FOOT ULCERS
Types of Ulcers

In general, ulcers can be divided into vascular/ischemic, neuropathic, or neuroischemic ulcers that make up the majority. It may be difficult to distinguish vascular from neuropathic ulcers as diabetes mellitus, when long-standing, tends to affect multiple organ systems. Peripheral neuropathy and peripheral arterial disease are also known to be significant independent risk factors for the development of diabetic foot ulcers and their recurrence.[16] **Table 2** shows typical features in terms of clinical appearance and examination results of the various ulcer types.[14]

Classification of Diabetic Foot Ulcers

DFUs can be described using a wide variety of classifications. The early established and most widely used classification is the Wagner or Wagner-Armstrong classification, which, however, is not sufficiently validated.[17] Monteiro-Soares and colleagues recommended that a classification should achieve 3 main clinical aims: to prognosticate, to facilitate communication between health professionals, and to facilitate clinical treatment decision-making. They evaluated 19 different classifications and concluded that currently, no classification sufficiently covers all 3 major purposes to be recommended.[17] The investigators, therefore, suggested using the site, ischemia, neuropathy, bacterial infection, area, and depth (SINBAD) score for communication between specialists and the Infectious Diseases Society of America/IWGDF criteria **(Table 3)** for documentation and infection classification purposes. The Wound-Ischemia-Foot-Infection (WIFI) classification score is useful for assessing vascular perfusion and identifying patients who may benefit from a revascularization intervention.[17]

Table 3
The International Working Group on the Diabetic Foot/Infectious Diseases Society of America classification of diabetic foot ulcer

Clinical Manifestations	Infection Severity	PEDIS Grade P = Perfusion E = Extension D = Depth I = Infection S = Sensation
Would lacking purulence or any manifestations of inflammation	Uninfected	1
Presence of more than or equal to 2 manifestation of inflammation (purulence or erythema, tenderness, warmth or induration), but any cellulitis/erythema extends ≤ 2 cm around the ulcer, and infection is limited to the skin or superficial subcutaneous tissues; no other local complications or systemic illness	Mild	2
Infection (as above) in a patient who is systemically well and metabolically stable but that has more than or equal to one of the following characteristics: cellulitis extending > 2 cm; lymphangitic streaking; spread beneath the superficial fascia; deep-tissue abscess; gangrene; and involvement of muscle, tendon, joint, or bone	Moderate	3
Infection in a patient with systemic toxicity or metabolic instability (eg,fever, chills, tachycardia, hypotension, confusion, vomiting, leukocytosis, acidosis, severe hyperglycemia, or azotemia)	Severe	4

Data from Lavery et al.[33]

The SINBAD classification consists of various parameters. One point is allocated for every parameter to a maximum count of 6 points. The classification contains the following parameters:[18]

- S = site, forefoot (0 points), mid- or hindfoot (1point)
- I = ischemia, at least one pulse palpable (0 points), clinical reduced pedal blood flow (1 point)
- N = neuropathy, detecting 10-g monofilament or Neurotip (0 points), no detection (1 point)
- B = bacterial infection, defined by IWGDF criteria if absent (0 points), present (1 point)
- A = area, less than 1 cm^2 (0 points), greater than 1 cm^2 (1 point)
- D = depth, skin or subcutaneous tissue (0 points), reaching muscle, tendon or deeper (1 point)

Identification of At-Risk Groups

The major aims of the IDFC are to identify those patients who are at risk for DFUs and of course to prevent the onset or progression of DFUs. Consequently, patients with an increased risk of DFUs should be thoroughly examined and followed-up closely. In addition, patients and relatives should be educated about the individual risk factors and how to modify these risk factors to reduce complications.[19] The basic clinical assessment is shown in **Table 4**.

Table 4 Basic examination of diabetic patients	
History	General history Foot history Foot symptoms
Physical examination	General examination Foot skin and footwear Neurologic examination Vascular examination
Auxiliary examination	Laboratory Ultrasound and electrophysical examination Imaging Pathologic and microbiological examination

ASSESSMENT OF THE MAIN RISK FACTORS FOR DIABETIC FOOT ULCERATION AND RISK CLASSIFICATION
Polyneuropathy

One of the most common risk factors for DFUs is peripheral polyneuropathy.[14] The relative risk of DFUs increases by a factor of 9 to 32 in the presence of polyneuropathy. Up to 78% of patients with diabetes mellitus suffer from polyneuropathy.[20] Typically, polyneuropathy caused by diabetes mellitus is mixed sensorimotor and shows symmetric distribution in both lower extremities. The natural course of polyneuropathy is progressive and irreversible. Clinical symptoms and test-based criteria can be used to diagnose peripheral polyneuropathy. Sensory neuropathy usually begins distally and can present with numbness, paresthesia, hypoesthesia, and dysesthesia and can also present with pain and allodynia. Motor neuropathy may present with muscle atrophy and motor deficits. The wasting of intrinsic foot muscles may result in muscle imbalances and may lead to forefoot deformities such as claw toes.[21] Autonomic neuropathy in the extremities causes sudomotor dysfunction and can present with dry skin, which is more susceptible to injury.[22] The standard examination should include the 10-g Semmes-Weinstein monofilament test, ankle reflexes, blunt/sharp, and warm/cold discrimination. Furthermore, vibration sensitivity should be tested with the 128-Hz tuning fork first at the metatarsophalangeal joint. If there is no sensation, then it should be tested at the medial malleolus.[23] Primary medical care providers can carry out these tests with little effort. If the monofilament and tuning fork are not available, a simpler light touch test can also help detect polyneuropathy.[11] Neurophysiological examinations with nerve-conduction-velocity measurements are still regarded as the gold standard for a sound diagnosis of peripheral polyneuropathy and provided in specialized departments. Muscle-nerve biopsies are usually not necessary in the case of polyneuropathy caused by diabetes mellitus but may be indicated for suspected hereditary neuromuscular disorders. A predominantly motor neuropathy, rapid development, asymmetry, involvement of cranial nerves, or beginning in the arms are atypical for diabetic polyneuropathy. In these cases, other diagnoses should be considered and ruled out by referring them to the relevant specialized departments for further assessment.[24]

Peripheral Arterial Disease

In addition to peripheral polyneuropathy, PAD and foot-intrinsic factors play a decisive role in the development of DFUs. PAD can occur in more than 50% of patients with DFU.[8] In up to 75% of diabetics with PAD, due to polyneuropathy, there are no typical

PAD symptoms such as claudication.[25] In diabetics with PAD, on top of progressive plaque formation in the intima of the arteries, medial artery sclerosis is also well known to be associated with diabetic PAD and is a useful indicator for a diabetic foot at risk.[26] After smoking, diabetes mellitus is the second most important risk factor for PAD. The risk of PAD is 2 to 4 times higher in diabetics than in the normal population. Compared with people without diabetes mellitus, PAD develops earlier in people with diabetes mellitus, progresses faster, and deteriorates more frequently into critical limb ischemia.[8]

The standard vascular diagnostics for diabetics include the following examinations[27,28]:

- Clinical examination with assessment of pedal pulse and capillary refill time
- Ultrasound ankle or toe pressure measurement (ankle brachial index [ABI], toe brachial index)
- Arterial duplex ultrasonography with pulse curve analysis

Other investigations to prognosticate include performing at least one of the following:

- Skin perfusion pressure measurement
- Toe pressure measurement
- Transcutaneous oxygen pressure measurement ($TcPO_2$)

An ABI greater than 0.7 (**Table 5**), a systolic ankle blood pressure greater than 70 mm Hg, and a systolic toe pressure greater than 40 mm Hg are required for appropriate wound healing. If these values are worse—ankle pressure less than 50 mm Hg, ABI less than 0.5, a toe pressure less than 30 mm Hg, or a $TcPO_2$ less than 25 mm Hg[28]—urgent vascular intervention should be considered, particularly, if the debridement- or amputation-wound does not heal.[1,8,28]

Further Intrinsic and Extrinsic Risk Factors

In addition to the 2 main risk factors, peripheral polyneuropathy and PAD, other intrinsic risk factors include altered foot anatomy and biomechanics and psychosocial factors.

The anatomy of the foot is altered due to polyneuropathy, which results in intrinsic muscle atrophy, wasting, and subsequently flexible or rigid claw-und hammertoe deformities. Increased glycosylation in soft tissues such as the Achilles tendon increases

Table 5 Ankle-brachial index	
Ankle-Brachial Index (ABI)	**Interpretation**
0.91–1.30	Normal
0.70–0.90	Mild obstruction
0.40–0.69	Intermediate obstruction
< 0.40	Severe obstruction
> 1.30	Incompressible, sclerotic arteries

Data from Hinchliffe et al.[28]

Table 6
Ulcer and amputation incidence based on The International Working Group on the Diabetic Foot risk classification

IWGDF Risk Classification	Incidence Ulcer (%)	Incidence Amputation (%)
0 Healthy foot	2	0.04
1 Polyneuropathy	3–4.5	0.7
2 Polyneuropathy and pAVKA	13.8	3.7
3 Previous ulcer or amputation	31.7	2.2
	32.2	20.7

Data from Lavery et al.[33]

its stiffness and limits ankle dorsiflexion[29–31] and increases stress on the forefoot. There is also increased stiffness in plantar soft tissues, which may also predispose the foot to ulceration.[31] Subsequently, abnormal pressure loads under the metatarsal heads in an insensate foot increase the risk of developing DFUs. Other causes of abnormal loading of the foot such as foot deformities, exostoses, or osteophytes can similarly lead to ulceration. These structural abnormalities may either be caused by diabetic-related cause such as muscle imbalances and Charcot's neuroarthropathy or may be caused by unrelated cause such as posttraumatic arthritis, degenerative arthritis, or congenital deformities. In some cases, the cause may be iatrogenic.[32]

Behavioral and psychological factors such as noncompliance, neglect, and depression are also among the intrinsic risk factors for DFUs.[27]

The extrinsic risk factors include inappropriate footwear, walking barefoot, or prolonged weight-bearing without consistent monitoring of the foot for calluses, blisters, or checking the footwear for foreign bodies. These extrinsic factors have a negative impact on the occurrence and healing of DFUs.[14]

International Working Group on the Diabetic Foot Risk Classification

The IWGDF recommends risk stratification of patients with DFU into 4 groups (**Table 6**). For group 0, which has no polyneuropathy and no PAD, an annual checkup of the foot by a trained specialist is sufficient to identify new risk factors and to be able to treat them accordingly. For Group 1 to 3 patients, there should be an increasing frequency of foot screening with increasing risk levels.[1] Approximately every third patient in the high-risk group will have another ulcer within 1 year, and the incidence for amputation in patients who had a previous amputation is 20% (see **Table 6**).[33]

THERAPY FOR DIABETIC FOOT ULCERS
Antibiotic Therapy

The DFU infections can either be monomicrobial or polymicrobial, with the latter being more common in chronic infections.[34] A recent meta-analysis by Macdonald and colleagues[35] showed that the spectrum of bacteria found is diverse, with *Staphylococcus aureus* being the most commonly isolated organism with the methicillin-resistant strain making up 18% of the total numbers. Other frequently isolated organisms are *Pseudomonas aeruginosa*, *Escherichia coli*, Proteus, and Enterococcus among others. Skin commensals are often detected in superficial microbiological samples, hence, adequate deep tissue biopsies for cultures and antibiotic sensitivity testing should be obtained to guide antibiotic treatment.[36] The choice of antibiotic therapy mainly depends on microbiological findings and antibiotic resistance. Before the organisms and their antibiotic sensitivities are reported, the SINBAD classification or the IWGDF guidelines can guide our choice of an appropriate empirical antibiotic regime.[36,37]

In the case of a superficial and stable DFU with decent granulation tissue and with no evidence of infection, antibiotic therapy is not indicated, and antiseptic wound dressings are usually sufficient. In the case of mild infections, oral antibiotics are prescribed for 1 to 2 weeks. In the case of high-grade infections with significant systemic and local signs of infection such as fever, tachycardia, hypotension, erythema, warmth, suppuration, wet gangrene, and with significantly deranged laboratory markers such as an elevated C-reactive protein and leukocyte count, admission is indicated. Early intravenous administration of antibiotics under close clinical and laboratory monitoring is recommended.[36,37]

Usually, the empirical administration of antibiotics according to each local hospital's guidelines is started immediately after tissue samples are taken for culture, and the therapy is adapted to the culture results and the antibiotic sensitivities. To avoid a rapidly ascending infection, empirical antibiotic therapy should be started as early as possible, when surgery with adequate biopsies is not possible within 6 to 12 hours. In the most of the cases, this early start of empirical antibiotics does not affect the microbiological diagnosis negatively due to poor vascularization of the diabetic feets. The benefit of preventing an ascending infection, septicemia, and its complications far outweigh the disadvantages of an inaccurate culture sample.

First-line antibiotics are usually clindamycin and/or third-generation cephalosporin or aminopenicillin. If anaerobic bacteria are suspected, metronidazole can be added.[36,37] Relevant secondary diseases such as kidney and liver diseases in diabetic patients must be considered, when choosing the antibiotic and the dosage. The dogma "time is tissue" should not be forgotten. Timely treatment can potentially save more tissue, increase the limb salvage rate, or at least diminish the extent of amputation.[38]

Offloading

Offloading of the affected limb is essential for the healing of a DFU and is best managed in close collaboration with either the orthotist, the shoe technician, or the podiatrist. For plantar ulcers, which are located in the forefoot or midfoot region, patients should be advised to either non–weight-bear or bear weight on their heels and be prescribed with a forefoot offloading shoe. The treatment regime depends greatly on the nature of the ulcer and the surgeon's assessment. If regular dressing changes are required, easily removable shoes or orthoses are worthwhile. For heel ulcers, patients are usually advised to non–weight-bear and may be prescribed a heel-off loading orthosis, which lowers regional pressure best and thus supports wound healing.[39] For offloading devices, there has been a paradigm shift away from using the total contact casts (TCC) to prefabricated knee-high orthoses, which can be made irremovable, such as the instant TCC. Second- and third-line recommendations include removable knee-high devices and removable ankle-high offloading devices, respectively. Some examples of knee-high devices include bivalved TCCs and knee-high walkers and examples of ankle-high devices include offloading shoes and cast shoes.[40] For DFUs that are nonplantar, ankle-high offloading devices such as a cast shoe or shoe modifications such as the addition of inner padding with padded dressings or altering the dimensions of the shoe and toe spacers should be considered, depending on the ulcer location.

Wound Therapy

The current IWGDF guideline[41] recommends debridement of all necrotic nonvital tissue in superficial and deep DFU unless there is dry necrosis. Surgical debridement should be repeated every 24 to 72 hours if new necrotic tissue arises and if there is still clinical and biochemical evidence of active infection. Negative pressure wound therapy (NPWT) to stimulate wound granulation and improve regional vascularization can be used postoperatively after surgical debridement. However, despite its increasing popularity, the current evidence of NPWT in improving wound healing rates and healing times is still weak. In the case of chronic ulcers, the benefit has not yet been scientifically proven.[41]

DFUs are not homogenous, and there is no "one-for-all" superior wound dressing. There is still an ambivalent study situation, when it comes to the use of specific wound dressings. Therefore, no recommendations should not be made at this point. However, important sound wound management principles should be emphasized.[14,27,41]

Keeping the wound environment optimized is crucial for successful wound treatment.[41] For a long time, the dogma of the dry wound environment was standard in DFU treatment. Except for removing excessive exudate, the dressing should maintain a moist environment to promote granulation and the subsequent healing process.[42] Dry necrosis should be kept dry. Otherwise, necrotic tissue should be removed frequently.[41]

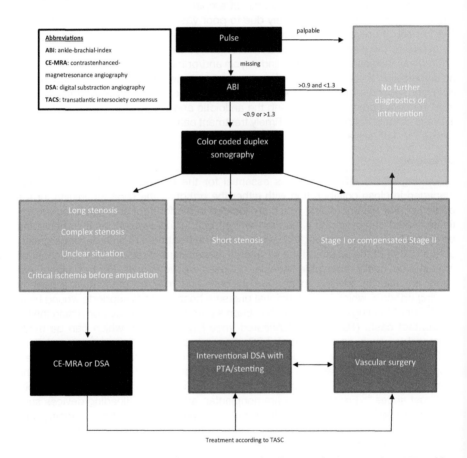

Fig. 1. Simplified diagnostic and therapeutic algorithm for vascular intervention. ABI, ankle-brachial-index; CE-MRA, contrastenhanced-magnetresonance angiography; DSA, digital substraction angiography; TACS, transatlantic intersociety consensus.S (*Data from* Rumenapf et al.[27])

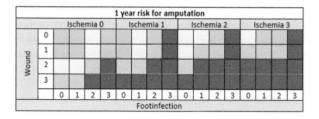

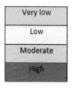

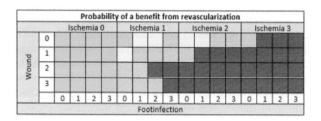

	W Wound	I Ischemia	fi Footinfection
0	No ulcer, no gangrene	ABI>0.8(pressure>100mmHg), TcPO2>60mmHg	No infection
1	Superficial ulcer, no gangrene	ABI<0.8(pressure<100mmHg), TcPO2<60mmHg	Mild infection: swelling, mild erythema, calor
2	Probe to bone/tendon/joint positive or forefoot gangrene	ABI<0.6(pressure<70mmHg), TcPO2<40mmHg	Local infection: erythema >2cm, subcutaneous structures involved
3	Massive ulcer or massive gangrene (for-, mid-, hindfoot)	ABI<0.4(pressure<50mmHg), TcPO2<30mmHg	Severe infection: Local infection with systemic signs SEPSIS, SIRS with

Fig. 2. The WIFI classification correlated with risk of amputation and probability of a benefit from revascularization. (*Data from* Rumenapf et al.[27])

Indications for Vascular Intervention

According to the IWGDF Guidelines,[28] no wound healing tendency within 4 to 6 weeks despite optimal management is an indication for further vascular imaging and revascularization. In addition, toe pressure less than 30 mm Hg, TcPO$_2$ less than 25 mm Hg, or ABI less than 0.5 are indications for urgent vascular imaging and intervention. Although ABI per se cannot be used as a prognostic factor for DFU healing, the amputation risk increases with an ABI less than 0.5 or ankle pressure less than 50 mm Hg.

A simplified diagnostic and therapeutic algorithm is shown in **Fig. 1.**

The WIFI classification is a prognostic tool to identify patients who may benefit from revascularization. It is divided into 3 main categories: wound grade, ischemia grade, and foot infection grade. **Fig. 2** shows the expected outcome of revascularization in the respective population ranging from very low benefit to high benefit.

In patients with DFU with symptomatic PAD, conservative treatment is recommended when there is either no strong indication for vascular intervention, the risk of intervention is too high, or intervention failed. The medical treatment regime includes the administration of antiplatelets (aspirin, 100 mg, or clopidogrel, 75 mg, daily) and the administration of statins and a structured vascular exercise program.[27,28]

PREVENTION OF DIABETIC FOOT ULCERS
Education for Patients and Relatives

Preventive education programs for patients and relatives are an integral part of the management of diabetes mellitus in many countries around the world and are well established. Although patient education to prevent DFUs has not been proved by randomized controlled trials,[43] individual studies report lower ulcer[44] and amputation rates.[14] Despite low-quality evidence, the IWGDF guidelines strongly support patient instruction not to walk barefoot, not to walk only in socks or thin slippers, and to wear suitable shoes made for diabetic feet lacking sensation. Furthermore, instruction of daily self-examination and regular self-care to prevent ulcers is recommended.[45] Some self-care strategies include keeping feet clean, ensuring skin between the toes is kept dry, using emollients to moisturize dry skin, and cutting toenails straight across.[11]

Shoe Wear

The consistent use of appropriate shoe wear should be checked at each clinical visit and incorporated into the patient education as well. Poorly fitting or inappropriate shoe wear may cause pressure concentration and repetitive trauma, which may lead to inflammation, soft tissue breakdown, and surprisingly rapid to DFU.[46] Diabetic polyneuropathy impairs not only the sensory but also the motor nerves and results in muscle imbalance of the foot. Common deformities due to muscle imbalance include equinus, hammertoes, claw toes, and even cavus feet.[47] These deformities are significant risk factors for DFU and also impede healing because of abnormal pressure concentration. For patients with deformities and who are at risk for ulceration, therapeutic shoes, custom-made insoles, or toe orthosis should be prescribed.[48] Off-the-shelf shoe wear with a wide toe box is sufficient for patients without severe foot deformity and polyneuropathy and thus with a low risk of DFU. However, regular reevaluation of the footwear and risk class is essential.[45]

Detection and Treatment of Preulcers

Prevention begins with the identification of preulcer lesions, which can manifest as hyperkeratosis, blisters, and infections. Regular monitoring and podiatry treatment with removal of the hyperkeratosis combined with various offloading modalities are recommended.[14] The relief of abnormal pressure areas reduces the risk of progression to DFUs.[45]

Preventive Surgical Measures and Perioperative Optimization

In the presence of foot deformities that cannot be adequately treated conservatively, surgical off-loading can be considered as a preventive measure.[45] The surgical techniques are wide-ranging, from flexor digitorum longus tenotomy in claw toes and exostectomies to complex reconstruction, for example, in severe deformities associated with Charcot arthropathy.[14,27] A surgical risk assessment should always be carried out before considering an elective surgical procedure. In addition to the usual surgical risks, asymptomatic PAD should be considered in order to avoid wound healing disorders.[27] Furthermore, perioperative hyper- and hypoglycemia should be avoided. Continuous glucose monitoring is of major importance to avoid those dysglycemic states and secondary complications.[49]

SUMMARY

Interdisciplinary treatment of diabetic patients ranging from basic local primary care to highly specialized IDFCs in tertiary hospitals should be the gold standard based on current evidence. A graded care team helps to triage patients with DFUs, optimizes medical resources, and reduces costs. Evaluation of team composition and improvement of the therapeutic and preventive algorithm should be the aim of further studies.

CLINICS CARE POINTS

- The interdisciplinary diabetic foot clinic (IDFC) should comprise of members with expertise in diabetic patient management working together on-site.

- The composition of IDFC cannot be generalised and should be optimised based on the individual hospital requirements, workflow, infrastructure and available expertise.

- The IDFC should have clinic-specific algorithms or pathways to help optimize each patient visit.

- The IDFC's access to various members of the interdisciplinary team should be readily available. For example, the infectious disease specialist for multidrug-resistant bacteria infection.

REFERENCES

1. Armstrong DG, Boulton AJM, Bus SA. Diabetic foot ulcers and their recurrence. N Engl J Med 2017;376:2367–75.
2. Zhang P, Lu J, Jing Y, et al. Global epidemiology of diabetic foot ulceration: a systematic review and meta-analysis. Ann Med (Helsinki) 2017;49:106–16.
3. Musuuza J, Sutherland BL, Kurter S, et al. A systematic review of multidisciplinary teams to reduce major amputations for patients with diabetic foot ulcers. J Vasc Surg 2020;71:1433–46.e3.
4. International Diabetes Federation. Time to act: diabetes and foot care. Brussels: International Diabetes Federation; 2005.
5. Armstrong DG, Kanda VA, Lavery LA, et al. Mind the gap: disparity between research funding and costs of care for diabetic foot ulcers. Diabetes care 2013;36:1815–7.
6. Rice JB, Desai U, Cummings AK, et al. Burden of diabetic foot ulcers for medicare and private insurers [published correction appears in Diabetes Care. Diabetes Care 2014;37(3):651–8.
7. Prompers L, Huijberts M, Apelqvist J, et al. High prevalence of ischaemia, infection and serious comorbidity in patients with diabetic foot disease in Europe. Baseline results from the Eurodiale study. Diabetologia 2007;50:18–25.
8. Rümenapf G, Morbach S, Rother U, et al. Diabetic foot syndrome-Part 1 : definition, pathophysiology, diagnostics and classification. Chirurg 2021;92:81.
9. Lipsky BA, Berendt AR, Cornia PB, et al. 2012 infectious diseases society of america clinical practice guideline for the diagnosis and treatment of diabetic foot infections. Clin Infect Dis 2012;54:e132–73.
10. Adiewere P, Gillis RB, Imran Jiwani S, et al. A systematic review and meta-analysis of patient education in preventing and reducing the incidence or recurrence of adult diabetes foot ulcers (DFU). Heliyon 2018;4:e00614.
11. Schaper NC, van Netten JJ, Apelqvist J, et al. Practical guidelines on the prevention and management of diabetic foot disease (IWGDF 2019 update). Diabetes Metab Res Rev 2020;36(Suppl 1):e3266.
12. Dutta A, Bhansali A, Rastogi A. Early and Intensive Glycemic Control for Diabetic Foot Ulcer Healing: A Prospective Observational Nested Cohort Study. Int J Lower Extremity Wounds 2021. https://doi.org/10.1177/15347346211033458.
13. Boyko EJ, Zelnick LR, Braffett BH, et al. Risk of foot ulcer and lower-extremity amputation among participants in the diabetes control and complications trial/

epidemiology of diabetes interventions and complications study. Diabetes care 2022;45:357–64.

14. Wang A, Lv G, Cheng X, et al. Guidelines on multidisciplinary approaches for the prevention and management of diabetic foot disease (2020 edition). Burns Trauma 2020;8:tkaa017.

15. Buggy A, Moore Z. The impact of the multidisciplinary team in the management of individuals with diabetic foot ulcers: a systematic review. J Wound Care 2017; 26(6):324–39.

16. Yazdanpanah L, Shahbazian H, Nazari I, et al. Incidence and risk factors of diabetic foot ulcer: a population-based diabetic foot cohort (ADFC Study)—two-year follow-up study. Int J Endocrinol 2018;2018:7631659-9.

17. Monteiro-Soares M, Boyko EJ, Jeffcoate W, et al. Diabetic foot ulcer classifications: a critical review. Diabetes Metab Res Rev 2020;36(Suppl 1):e3272.

18. Ince P, Abbas ZG, Lutale JK, et al. Use of the SINBAD classification system and score in comparing outcome of foot ulcer management on three continents. Diabetes Care 2008;31(5):964–7.

19. Sorber R, Abularrage CJ. Diabetic foot ulcers: Epidemiology and the role of multidisciplinary care teams. Semin Vasc Surg Mar 2021;34(1):47–53.

20. Boulton AJ, Kirsner RS, Vileikyte L. Clinical practice. Neuropathic diabetic foot ulcers. N Engl J Med 2004;351(1):48–55.

21. Bus SA, Yang QX, Wang JH, et al. Intrinsic muscle atrophy and toe deformity in the diabetic neuropathic foot: a magnetic resonance imaging study. Diabetes Care 2002;25:1444–50.

22. Tentolouris N, Marinou K, Kokotis P, et al. Sudomotor dysfunction is associated with foot ulceration in diabetes. Diabetic Med 2009;26:302–5.

23. Volmer-Thole M, Lobmann R. Neuropathy and Diabetic Foot Syndrome. Int J Mol Sci 2016;17:917.

24. Heuß, D. S1-Leitlinie: Diagnostik bei Polyneuropathien. *DGNeurologie* 2, 2019; 359–82.

25. Balletshofer B, Ito W, Lawall H, et al. Position paper on the diagnosis and treatment of peripheral arterial disease (PAD) in people with diabetes mellitus. Exp Clin Endocrinol Diabetes 2019;127(S 01):S105–13.

26. David Smith C, Gavin Bilmen J, Iqbal S, et al. Medial artery calcification as an indicator of diabetic peripheral vascular disease. Foot Ankle Int 2008;29(2):185–90.

27. Rümenapf G, Morbach S, Rother U, et al. Diabetic foot syndrome-Part 2 : revascularization, treatment alternatives, care structures, recurrency prophylaxis. Chirurg 2021;92:173–86.

28. Hinchliffe RJ, Forsythe RO, Apelqvist J, et al. Guidelines on diagnosis, prognosis, and management of peripheral artery disease in patients with foot ulcers and diabetes (IWGDF 2019 update). Diabetes Metab Res Rev 2020;36(Suppl 1):e3276.

29. Singh VP, Bali A, Singh N, et al. Advanced glycation end products and diabetic complications. Korean J Physiol Pharmacol 2014;18:1–14.

30. Rao SR, Saltzman CL, Wilken J, et al. Increased passive ankle stiffness and reduced dorsiflexion range of motion in individuals with diabetes mellitus. Foot Ankle Int 2006;27(8):617–22.

31. Khor BYC, Woodburn J, Newcombe L, et al. Plantar soft tissues and Achilles tendon thickness and stiffness in people with diabetes: a systematic review. J Foot Ankle Res 2021;14:35.

32. Rogers LC, Andros G, Caporusso J, et al. Toe and flow: essential components and structure of the amputation prevention team. J Vasc Surg 2010;52(3 Suppl):23S–7S.

33. Lavery LA, La Fontaine J, Kim PJ. Preventing the first or recurrent ulcers. Med Clin North Am 2013;97(5):807–20.
34. Kwon KT, Armstrong DG. Microbiology and antimicrobial therapy for diabetic foot infections. Infect Chemother 2018;50(1):11–20.
35. Macdonald KE, Boeckh S, Stacey HJ, et al. The microbiology of diabetic foot infections: a meta-analysis. BMC Infect Dis 2021;21(1):770.
36. Lipsky BA, Senneville E, Abbas ZG, et al. Guidelines on the diagnosis and treatment of foot infection in persons with diabetes (IWGDF 2019 update). Diabetes Metab Res Rev 2020;36(Suppl 1):e3280.
37. Hingorani A, LaMuraglia GM, Henke P, et al. The management of diabetic foot: A clinical practice guideline by the Society for Vascular Surgery in collaboration with the American Podiatric Medical Association and the Society for Vascular Medicine. J Vasc Surg 2016;63(2 Suppl):3S–21S. https://doi.org/10.1016/j.jvs.2015.10.003.
38. Vas PRJ, Edmonds M, Kavarthapu V, et al. The Diabetic Foot Attack: "'Tis Too Late to Retreat. Int J Lower Extremity Wounds 2018;17(1):7–13.
39. Bus SA, Armstrong DG, Gooday C, et al. Guidelines on offloading foot ulcers in persons with diabetes (IWGDF 2019 update). Diabetes Metab Res Rev 2020;36(Suppl 1):e3274.
40. Lazzarini PA, Jarl G. Knee-high devices are gold in closing the foot ulcer gap: a review of offloading treatments to heal diabetic foot ulcers. Medicina (Kaunas) 2021;57(9):941.
41. Rayman G, Vas P, Dhatariya K, et al. Guidelines on use of interventions to enhance healing of chronic foot ulcers in diabetes (IWGDF 2019 update). Diabetes Metab Res Rev 2020;36(Suppl 1):e3283.
42. Everett E, Mathioudakis N. Update on management of diabetic foot ulcers. Ann N Y Acad Sci 2018;1411(1):153–65.
43. Lincoln NB, Radford KA, Game FL, et al. Education for secondary prevention of foot ulcers in people with diabetes: a randomised controlled trial. Diabetologia 2008;51(11):1954–61.
44. Calle-Pascual AL, Duran A, Benedi A, et al. Reduction in foot ulcer incidence: relation to compliance with a prophylactic foot care program. Diabetes Care 2001;24(2):405–7.
45. Bus SA, Lavery LA, Monteiro-Soares M, et al. Guidelines on the prevention of foot ulcers in persons with diabetes (IWGDF 2019 update). Diabetes Metab Res Rev 2020;36(Suppl 1):e3269.
46. Frykberg RG, Wukich DK, Kavarthapu V, et al. Surgery for the diabetic foot: a key component of care. Diabetes Metab Res Rev 2020;36(Suppl 1):e3251.
47. Frykberg RG, Bevilacqua NJ, Habershaw G. Surgical off-loading of the diabetic foot. J Vasc Surg 2010;52(3 Suppl):44s–58s.
48. Bus SA, Armstrong DG, van Deursen RW, et al. IWGDF guidance on footwear and offloading interventions to prevent and heal foot ulcers in patients with diabetes. Diabetes Metab Res Rev 2016;32(Suppl 1):25–36.
49. Ehrenfeld JM, Wanderer JP, Terekhov M, et al. A perioperative systems design to improve intraoperative glucose monitoring is associated with a reduction in surgical site infections in a diabetic patient population. Anesthesiology 2017;126(3):431–40.

Distal Metatarsal Osteotomies for Chronic Plantar Diabetic Foot Ulcers

Carlo Biz, MD[a,b,*], Pietro Ruggieri, MD, PhD[a]

KEYWORDS

- Diabetic foot • Diabetic ulcer • Distal metatarsal osteotomies • Metatarsalgia
- Minimally invasive surgery • Neuropathic ulcers • Percutaneous surgery

KEY POINTS

- Currently, distal metatarsal osteotomies (DMOs) represent the successful application of the best principles of minimally invasive surgery, historically used for the treatment of metatarsalgia, in the operative management of chronic plantar diabetic foot ulcers (CPDFUs).
- DMOs, performed at a different level of the distal metatarsal bones, reduce the pressure on the CPDFU and promote its healing.
- These percutaneous osteotomies (DMOs), planned correctly using weight-bearing dorso-plantar radiographs of the diabetic foot, can restore the original harmonic distal parabola of the forefoot and/or create a new balanced forefoot arch, preventing ulcer recurrence.
- DMOs are completely changing the traditional surgical approach to CPDFUs with osteo-myelitis, preserving the infected metatarsal bone as much as possible.
- The recent literature has proven DMOs to be a safe and effective method for the operative management of CPDFUs, regardless of their severity.

INTRODUCTION

Chronic plantar diabetic foot ulcers (CPDFUs) are common among diabetic patients (DPs), with a reported annual incidence of 2% to 6%.[1-4] Those at the level of the metatarsal heads (MHs) are common and represent 22% of all foot ulcers.[5] It has been estimated that approximately 25% of hospitalizations are directly related to foot problems,[6] which are responsible for nearly 50% of the hospital bed days caused

[a] Orthopedics and Orthopedic Oncology, Department of Surgery, Oncology and Gastroenterology DiSCOG, University of Padova, Via Giustiniani 2, Padova 35128, Italy; [b] Minimally Invasive Foot and Ankle Society (MIFAS by GRECMIP), 2 Rue Georges Negrevergne, Merignac 33700, France
* Corresponding author. Orthopedics and Orthopedic Oncology, Department of Surgery, Oncology and Gastroenterology DiSCOG, University of Padova, Via Giustiniani 2, Padova 35128, Italy.
E-mail address: carlo.biz@unipd.it

Foot Ankle Clin N Am 27 (2022) 545–566
https://doi.org/10.1016/j.fcl.2022.02.003
1083-7515/22/© 2022 Elsevier Inc. All rights reserved.

by diabetes,[7] whereas the lifetime risk of developing diabetic foot ulcers (DFUs) is estimated around 19% to 34%.[8] More than half of these lesions become infected, and approximately 15% to 20% of them lead to some level of amputation (**Fig. 1**).[9,10] Furthermore, DPs with pressure ulcers have a 2.5-fold increased risk of death compared with the same patients without CPDFUs.[11] Specifically, CPDFU development is associated with 5% mortality during the first year and 42% mortality within 5 years.[11] It is not surprising that the National Health Service in England spends over £1 billion annually managing DFUs and their consequences, which accounts for ~10% of the National Health Service diabetes budget.[12]

The development of CPDFUs is frequently correlated with the following 4 major factors:[13] *(1) peripheral neuropathy* (insensate foot); *(2) vascular disease; (3) elevated local pressure under the MHs* due to a plantarflexion deformity of one or more of the metatarsal bones (MBs), and also to hyperextension of the proximal phalanx (P1) when claw toe deformity is present;[14–18] and *(4) the tendency of plantar tissue in DPs to be stiffer than the one in healthy subjects*, developing more intense stress-relaxation phenomena.[19] These factors lead to hypertrophic callus formation and increased risk for local ulcers (**Fig. 2**).[20]

With appropriate conservative therapy, including antibiotics when necessary, surgical debridement, off-loading of pressure, attention to infection, and if necessary, vascular reconstruction, foot ulcers heal in many patients, and the need for amputation is averted.[21,22] At present, total contact casting is still the most popular offloading method of treating these ulcers.[23–25] However, for diabetic neuropathic patients, we believe that the restriction of complete non–weight bearing is impractical, harmful, and illusory.

Unfortunately, even after the resolution of a DFU, the recurrence rate is 40% following the first year aftercare and starting full weight bearing, 60% within the first 3 years, and 65% within 5 years.[20] For this reason, as suggested by Tamir and colleagues,[26] even after successful of the conservative management described and its maintenance by appropriate local treatment and shoe modifications, the DFU *"is not considered cured but is more appropriately termed as in remission."*[26–28]

Currently, in case of failure of conservative management, the application of minimally invasive surgery (MIS) in the treatment of recalcitrant ulcers,[6] which has become quite popular among foot surgeons during the past decade because of its several

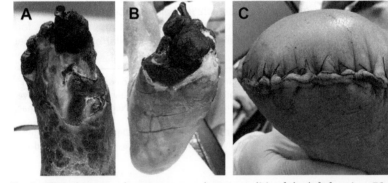

Fig. 1. *Clinical images:* dry gangrene and osteomyelitis of the left foot in a 76-year-old diabetic man with severe peripheral arterial disease and previous CPDFUs becoming infected (*A, B*) and leading to a midthigh amputation (*C*).

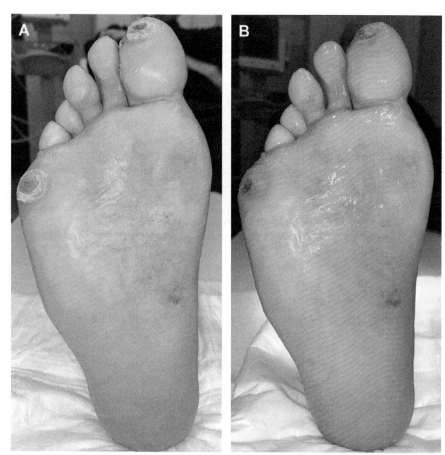

Fig. 2. *Clinical images*: a 54-year-old diabetic man, presenting hypertrophic callus formations at the level of the fifth MH and distal phalanx of the big toe in his right foot (*A*), masking plantar DFUs (*B*).

advantages (no tourniquet, minimal surgical scars and tissue damage, immediately postoperative weight bearing),[29,30] represents a successful new strategy. This is also because the traditional operative methods, including both bone procedures and tendon balancing,[31–33] are often correlated with high complication rates, such as infections and wound recurrences.[34–36]

In this report, we intend to promote the use of DMOs for the resolution of CPDFUs, which allow us to apply the already well-known and appreciated features of MIS to the lesions, even chronic, of the diabetic forefoot, achieving their healing by a better distribution of plantar pressure on the MB (Maestro criteria) and without internal fixation (giving lower infection risk).

Purpose of DMOs

Different minimally invasive and percutaneous distal metatarsal osteotomies (DMOs) at different levels of the distal MB have been proposed in more than 30 years (1986–2022).[24] However, they have 2 main common goals:

1. favoring the reduction of bone-induced pressure on the CPDFUs to consequently promote their healing;
2. restoring the metatarsal parabola of the forefoot, preventing recurrent transfer skin lesions and possible future wound and bone infection.[37]

ESSENTIAL FEATURES OF DMOs AND THEIR HISTORICAL PERSPECTIVE

From 1986 to the present, relatively few original studies regarding DMOs for CPDFUs have been published proposing different osteotomy shapes.[26,38–43] Despite the heterogeneity of the surgical procedures described, the different authors showed a systematic, minimally invasive, common approach to the management of diabetic ulcers.
All DMOs were:

- performed in a minimally invasive way;
- carried out by an incision smaller than 3 cm;
- performed by a foot dorsal approach at the level of the lesser distal MBs;
- drawn down in oblique slide shape;
- never fixed (if not temporary, using K-wires).

DMOs Procedures Proposed (1986–2021)

- *1986:* Wray and colleagues[43] described a metatarsal neck osteotomy of the MBs **(Fig. 3A)**, osteotomized obliquely, starting proximally on the dorsum but proceeding distally and plantar-ward at an angle of 45°.
- *1990:* Tillo and colleagues[42] **(Fig. 3B)** proposed 4 different types of DMOs: osteoclasis of the MH (B1), V-osteotomy, shortening colectomy (B2), and oblique slide osteotomy (B3).
- *2016:* Tamir and colleagues[40] **(Fig. 3C)** used a perpendicular or short oblique osteotomy performed at the neck or diaphysis of the MB.

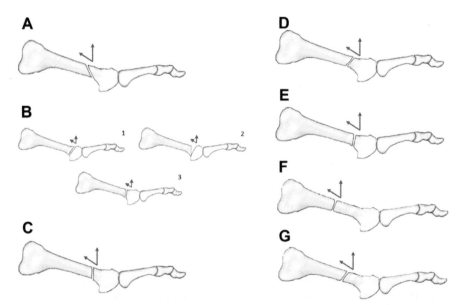

Fig. 3. Different shapes of DMOs (*A–G*) proposed by several authors from 1986 to 2021.

- *2018:* Biz and colleagues[38] (**Fig. 3**D) proposed a distal metatarsal diaphyseal osteotomy performed with an angle of approximately 45° with respect to the long axis of the lesser MB in a dorsal-distal to proximal-plantar direction.
- *2020:* Similarly, Tamir and colleagues[41] (**Fig. 3**E) treated another series of patients using a DMO perpendicular to the first MB distal metaphysis.
- *2020:* In the same year, Chiu and colleagues[39] (**Fig. 3**F) proposed a distal diaphyseal ostectomy proximal to the level of the metatarsal neck to preserve also metatarsophalangeal joint (MTPJ) function.
- *2021:* Tamir and colleagues[26] (**Fig. 3**G) described a minimally invasive floating distal metatarsal oblique osteotomy.

INDICATIONS AND CONTRAINDICATIONS
Indications

DMOs are indicated when:

- conservative methods fail, usually after at least 6 weeks of off-loading orthotic treatment using total contact cast (most popular but not preferable method), removable walking boot, corrective shoes with a customized insole (both preferable), and standard conservative treatment including medications.[44]
- in situations where there is poor local soft tissue or previous amputations of toes and/or MBs with scarring.
- the presence of significant arthritis and stiffness in the associated MTPJ and the consequent association of reported increased risk of nonunion in this situation[44,45] is not a contraindication for DMO, as it is a diaphyseal osteotomy.

Relative Contraindications (Perform DMO with Caution-Selected Cases)

- Ulcers with chronic infection or ulcers penetrating deep structures;
- osteomyelitis of the MBs or the phalanges;
- ankle-brachial index below 0.5 and flat pulse volume recording at the ankle level (discuss case with vascular surgeon).

Absolute Contraindications

- Severe ischemia;
- gangrene, defined in the International Consensus on the Diabetic Foot as a continuous necrosis of the skin and the underlying structures (muscle, tendon, joint, or bone).
- extensive soft tissue infection of the forefoot;
- cellulitis of the foot or toe.

CLINICAL PREOPERATIVE EVALUATION AND RADIOGRAPHIC PLANNING
Clinical Aspects

In treating CPDFUs, both clinical and radiological assessments are mandatory for preoperative planning. The general aspects of the diabetic foot (DF) with related ulcerations and patient's clinical condition, including control of blood sugar, must be evaluated, as previously reported by these authors:[37]

- affected side;
- site of plantar lesion;
- depth and size of the ulcer;
- clinical signs of infection and dorsal dislocation of P1.

Ulcer Classification

The University of Texas Diabetic Wound Classification System (UTDWC)[46,47] is routinely used to grade CPDFUs (**Table 1**), whereas the ulcer's diameter and the major axes of the wounds can be determined manually using a transparent sheet, as originally described by Coughlin,[48] or more simply by a ruler.

Planning

The number of DMOs that must be performed in each forefoot is planned according to how much the metatarsal formula is altered, following the Maestro criteria.[38,49] These criteria quantify the levels of disorders of harmony of the forefoot and the metatarsal length, which are the cause of progressive skin lesions until ulceration.[35] For this reason, the following radiographic criteria must be evaluated on the preoperative weight-bearing radiographs (**Fig. 4**: *case 1*), as we previously described:[38]

- M1M2 index;
- Maestro 1 (M1);
- Maestro 2 (M2);
- Maestro 3 (M3).

This allows making the decision (see **Fig. 4**A) where the DMOs should be performed to achieve the following surgical goals (with a tolerance of ± 1 mm for Maestro criteria 1 and 2, ± 2 mm for Maestro criteria 3)[38,49]:

- to rebalance plantar pressures;
- to create a harmonious curve (parabola);
- to promote and maintain ulcer healing over time (see **Fig. 4**B–D).

Note that a DMO should be carried out only on the MH causing the plantar lesion unless this shortening would make the neighboring MB too long, resulting in a disharmonious morphotype with a high risk of a transfer plantar lesion. The adjacent MB must be also shortened in this case (see **Fig. 4**A–C).

THE OPERATIVE ASPECTS OF THE DMO TECHNIQUE
Equipment

For a correct operative procedure, the following are necessary:

- a small scalpel blade (SM64);
- periosteal elevator and bone rasp;
- a Shannon Isham burr (2.0 × 12 mm);
- a 20-cc syringe with normal saline solution;
- a fluoroscopy system for radiographic check;
- a power-driven burr, which has to provide a speed of approximately 2000 to 6000 rpm to avoid bone necrosis;
- bandages and tubular gauze for the final dressing.

Regional Ultrasound-Guided Anesthesia

According to the anesthetist's experience, 2 different types of ultrasound-guided regional anesthesia are recommended:

- sciatic-femoral block;
- ankle-block.

To improve patient cooperation and comfort:

Table 1
The University of Texas Diabetic Wound Classification (UTDWC) used to grade CPDFUs.[46,47]

Ulcer	Grade			
Stage	0	I	II	III
A	Preulcerative or postulcerative lesion completely epithelialized	Superficial wound, not involving tendon, capsule, or bone	Wound penetrating to tendon or capsule	Wound penetrating to bone or joint
B	Preulcerative or postulcerative lesion completely epithelialized with infection	Superficial wound, not involving tendon, capsule, or bone with infection	Wound penetrating to tendon or capsule with infection	Wound penetrating to bone or joint with infection
C	Preulcerative or postulcerative lesion completely epithelialized with ischemia	Superficial wound, not involving tendon, capsule, or bone with ischemia	Wound penetrating to tendon or capsule with ischemia	Wound penetrating to bone or joint with ischemia
D	Preulcerative or postulcerative lesion completely epithelialized with infection and ischemia	Superficial wound, not involving tendon, capsule, or bone with infection and ischemia	Wound penetrating to tendon or capsule with infection and ischemia	Wound penetrating to bone or joint with infection and ischemia

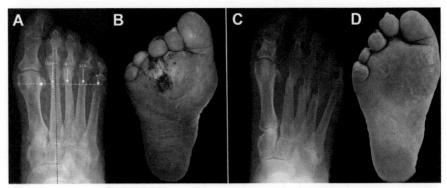

Fig. 4. *Case 1:* a 76-year-old diabetic female patient having undergone DMDO of the second, third, and fourth MB for a CPDFU (II B, UTDWC) and percutaneous osteotomy of P1 of the first, second, and third toes associated to percutaneous tenotomy procedures for claw deformity. Radiographic marks, measurements and M1M2 index according to Maestro criteria on the anteroposterior weight-bearing radiograph during surgical planning to calculate the number of MBs to shorten (*A*) and identification of the ulcer at the level of the 4MH on the plantar aspect of her foot at preoperative period (*B*). Radiographic and clinical images at 18-month follow-up, showing a more harmonious forefoot morphotype, bone callus consolidation of percutaneous osteotomies performed (*C*), and the conservation of complete healing of the ulcer, which was reached after 3 months from MIS (*D*).

- standard premedication should be administered using intravenous midazolam (1–2 mg) and fentanyl (0.1 mg);
- intraoperative sedation is obtained using propofol 1.5 mg/kg to 2.5 mg/kg for initiation and a continuous infusion of 4–8 mg/kg/h for maintenance.[50]

Positioning During the Operation

- The patient is in a supine position with the operated DF protruding from the table;
- the C-arm is positioned under the foot for direct and continuous control of the procedure;
- no ankle joint tourniquet is applied for two reasons:
  - blood is necessary to facilitate the removal of bone debris to be eliminated in the form of bone paste;
  - and more importantly, it is not indicated in diabetic lower limb surgery because of the compromised vascular peripheral system.

Surgical Technique

The surgical technique is performed according to the same principles and the same general indications previously described.[37,38] Here it is described for a CPDFU in a left foot (**Fig. 5**).

- *Portals:* the top of the MH must first be palpated with the left thumb. Then, moving a few millimeters proximally at this level in the interspace on the right side of the MH, an incision of 5 mm is made parallel to the extensor tendons with a small scalpel blade (SM64), held by the dominant hand of the surgeon, at the dorsal side of the medial border of each MH that needs to be shortened. The side of the incision depends on whether the surgeon is right- or left-handed and which foot is being operated on.

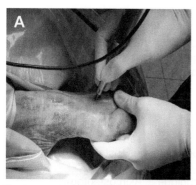
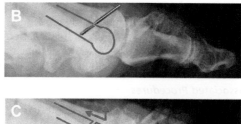
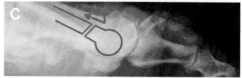

Fig. 5. *Surgical technique.* A DMO is performed by a 12-mm Shannon Isham burr with an angle of approximately 45° with respect to the long axis of the lesser MB in a dorsal-distal to proximal-plantar direction (*A*). Lateral view radiographs of a left DF on weight bearing before (*B*) and after (*C*) the osteotomy performed proximal to the neck with potentially greater elevation of MH from the ground.

- *Osteotomy site:* the scalpel is moved forward at an oblique angle of about 45° until it reaches the dorsal aspect of the distal MB, proximal to the neck, to undergo osteotomy. Through the same incision, first a bone rasp is inserted, and the periosteum is separated at the level of the osteotomy. A path is then prepared for the burr by using a periosteal elevator and positioning it obliquely at a 45° angle to the metatarsal axis, against the neck. This can be done by feel, using the instrument to move along the flare on the proximal part of the neck, from neck to distal diaphysis, mirroring the movement needed then for the osteotomy and detaching the tissues, which tend to be very stiff in diabetic feet.
- *Osteotomy:* a Shannon Isham burr (2.0 × 12 mm) is introduced until it reaches the metatarsal neck. It is then retracted a few millimeters proximally where the periosteum was previously removed (see **Fig. 5**A). Fluoroscopy allows confirmation of the correct position of the osteotomy site on the distal diaphysis of the MB. In this position, cutting is started with an angle of approximately 45° with respect to the long axis of the MB in a dorsal-distal to proximal-plantar direction, with rotary motion, extending to the contralateral cortex. The lateral or medial cortical surface, respectively, for left or right foot, is cut first in this way, followed by the plantar, medial, or lateral, and lastly, the dorsal cortical surface. Beginning with the section of the lateral cortex, the osteotomy is started with the motorized burr moving in a plantar and medial direction and ends with the section of the dorsal cortex. This is carried out by pivoting in a rotational movement from the point of skin entry, involving a supination of the wrist of 90°. Thus, the burr comes to lie nearly flat on the foot at 90° to the metatarsal axis in the anteroposterior plane.
- *Portal irrigation:* the incision site is irrigated by normal saline during osteotomy because the burr can cause excessive heat, first burning the skin and subsequently resulting in fibrosis and pseudoarthrosis at the bone level.[29,44,51] The lavage is also useful to remove bone debris, preventing periarticular ossifications in the stab canal.
- *Compacting of osteotomy sides:* the bone is manually compacted upon completion of the osteotomy by exercising pressure in the distal-proximal direction,

pushing the MH dorsally and producing contact of the trabecular bone since no internal fixation is performed (see **Fig.** 5B, C).
- *Ulcer debridement:* by accurate ulcer debridement, the CPDFU is converted into an acute wound to enable the normal stages of healing: primary, when wound closure is possible by suture; secondary, in other cases.[52,53]

Associated Procedures

In the cases of associated hallux valgus (HV) or claw toe deformity, with or without ulcers, the local forefoot surgery protocol is followed, for:

- mild to moderate HV: Reverdin-Isham percutaneous osteotomy, +/− Akin osteotomy;[29,45]
- moderate to severe HV: MIND/Endolog technique ± Akin osteotomy;[29,44,54]
- toe *deformities:* surgical algorithm as described by Redfern and Vernois.[45]

These additional procedures must be planned in the same operation with extreme caution according to the vascular condition of the foot. For all, there are the same relative and absolute contraindications described previously for DMOs, except for the Endolog Technique involving a minimally invasive intramedullary nail in which the relative ones have to be considered absolute.[54,55]

Bandage

Because no internal fixation is performed in this surgery, the bandage is very important to maintain the MH position achieved after DMO. A surgeon wishing to attempt these techniques must be familiar with the proper wrapping of the bandage to control the MB axis and toe position in the postoperative period while healing occurs.

After having covered the debrided ulcer with gauze, it is useful to use:

- *tape for bandages,* bent and crisscrossed, tracing between all intermetatarsal spaces, crossing them over the medial (lateral) aspect of each of the osteotomies performed (depending on the foot side) to reinforce the strength of the bandage;
- *gentle traction* to maintain the toe in slight plantar inclination (if possible);
- *tubular gauze* to cover the forefoot, except for the distal part of the toes and nails to check distal vascularization of the foot.

Postoperative Care

According to our postoperative protocol:

- *Day 0:* before the DP's discharge, anteroposterior and lateral radiographs of non–weight-bearing feet should be taken.
- *Days 1 to 7:* oral antibiotic prophylaxis for a week is recommended starting from the day of the surgery.
- *Days 1 to 30:* thromboembolic prophylaxis (Natrium enoxaparin: 4000 IU/day) and an antiedema therapy (Leucoselect, Lymphaselect, and Bromelain: 1 cp/day) are prescribed for 30 days. Furthermore, an analgesic therapy is advised in the morning for only 2 weeks using etoricoxib, 60 mg, 1 cp/day (when comorbidities of the DP permit it), also to prevent heterotopic ossification; or alternatively, paracetamol (1 g, 1 cp x2/d). During the first month, the DPs are allowed to walk using a rigid flat-soled orthopedic shoe for the following 30-day period. This is very important as metatarsal length is set automatically upon weight bearing of the foot.
- *Days 7 to 30:* each of the DPs is seen once a week for a month on an outpatient basis. The first control is 8 days after surgery. The original bandage is removed

and substituted by a simpler bandage. At the next 3 weekly visits, the bandage is changed in the same way.

- *Day 30:* The bandage is totally removed 1 month after surgery if the ulcer is completely closed, and anteroposterior weight-bearing and lateral radiographs are taken. The patient is then able to walk with comfortable shoes; or orthopedic footwear usually used (according to previous DF deformity); or new orthosis (if the foot deformity has been improved after the operation), allowing total load on the operated foot. If the CPDFU is not completely healed, the patient is seen every week for medication until total healing of the lesion.

CLINICAL OUTCOMES

Reliable scientific evidence is essential to guide the use of the MIS in clinical practice applied to the diabetic feet for the management of CPDFUs. Overall, the studies presented in the literature report encouraging and promising results following DMOs regarding:

- ulcer healing (range 55.1%–100.0%);
- mean healing time (range from 1 to 2 months);
- recurrence rates (range 0.0% to 13.6%).

In the study by Tamir and colleagues[40] (2016), 17 of 20 lesions (85.0%) completely healed, whereas the remaining 3 of 20 lesions (15.0%) improved. If we consider other studies, the healing rate was greater than 90.0% and the healing time reported ranged from 1 to 2 months.[26,38–43]

In our previous series of 30 patients, preoperative AOFAS score was computed at 55.3 ± 8.3 (range 42–71),[38] whereas AOFAS at last follow-up was 81.4 ± 9.1 (range 64–100). Postoperative VAS for satisfaction was computed at 9.8 ± 0.7 (range 7–10).[38]

More recently, Tamir and colleagues[26] reported the peak pressure under the head of the osteotomized MB. This outcome was found to decrease from 338.1 to 225.4 kPa (33%, $P < .0001$) after surgery; the pressure-time integral under the osteotomized MH decreased as well from 82.4 kPa to 65.0 kPa s (21%, $P < .0001$).[26]

Challenging Clinical Case: DMOs for Ulcerated Charcot Foot

A 71-year-old male patient with a long medical history of type II diabetes and peripheral distal neuropathy was seen in the multidisciplinary DF clinic at our institution for a second opinion *(Case 2)*. He presented a wide soft-tissue lesion (IIIB, UTDWC[46,47]) in the plantar region of his left Charcot foot (**Fig. 6A, B**), involving all of the MTPJs of the lesser MBs (second to fifth), associated with other midfoot and calcaneal DFUs (IA, UTDWC[46,47]). The DFU initially appeared 9 months before, becoming bigger over time, and he had been unable to walk in the last 4 months, routinely using a wheelchair. As the previous treatment failed at another institution, a below-knee amputation was suggested, which the patient refused. For the patient's inability to stand up, non–weight-bearing radiographs were taken (**Fig. 6C, D**), and a 2D-3D CT scan was performed (**Fig. 7A, B**).

Surgery was planned after 2 months of weekly visits for change of dressing and local debridement (**Fig. 7C**). In association with hyperbaric oxygen therapy and prolonged necessary refraining from walking, this allowed not only to conservatively resolve the associated minor DFUs and a further ulcer on the first toe that appeared during the follow-up (**Fig. 7D**) but also to reduce the major plantar lesion (**Fig. 8A, B**). Based on clinical and radiographic images, the DP underwent DMO of the second, third, fourth, and fifth MB (**Fig. 8C; Fig. 9B–D**). After surgery, the patient was allowed to

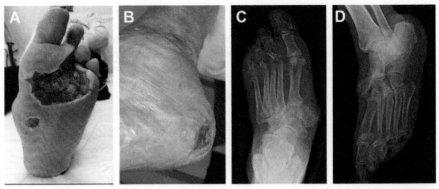

Fig. 6. *Case 2:* clinical (*A, B*) and radiographic images (*C, D*) of the ulcerated left Charcot foot at the time of DP's presentation.

walk using a rigid flat-soled orthopedic shoe and crutches. Subsequently, the major CPDFU was progressively reduced (**Fig. 9**A–C) until complete clinical and radiographic healing at 10 months from the operation (**Fig. 10**B–E), and the patient resumed normal walking after a month of physical therapy (**Fig. 10**A).

Complications of DMOs

DMOs show an overall complication range between 44.9% and 68.2%. The most common complications reported in the literature in order of frequency are:

- *Foot swelling (56.3%)*

It is generally persistent and moderate, affecting the forefoot for more than 6 weeks without infection, which improves after some months with complete callus formation at the osteotomy sites and without further treatment.[24,38]

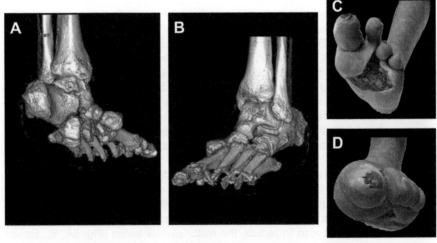

Fig. 7. *Case 2:* 3D CT scan Charcot foot images: posterior and anterior views (*A, B*), respectively. Clinical images after soft-tissue debridement sections (*C, D*).

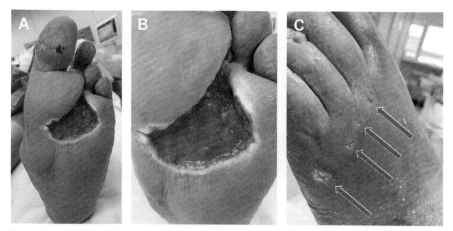

Fig. 8. *Case 2:* clinical images of the Charcot foot at the time of surgery showing the reduction of the plantar lesion after conservative treatment, the healing of the associated ulcers (IA, UTDWC[46,47]) (*A, B*), and the 3-mm portals on the dorsal aspect of the left foot (*red arrows*) through which DMOs were performed on the second to fifth MBs (*C*).

- *Radiographic nonunion (4.5%-30.0%)*

Fortunately, it is often described as asymptomatic probably because of the sensory neuropathy of these patients.[26,40,41]

- *Infections (4.2%-25.2%)*

Infections often adversely affect the healing of plantar DFUs. Usually, they are mainly superficial and treated successfully with oral or intravenous antibiotics. However, when exceptionally deep infections appear, subsequent surgical treatment is mandatory.[26,38–41] When fixation is used to prevent nonunion, using temporary K-wires or cancellous bone screws, a higher infection rate (31.8%) has been reported.[56]

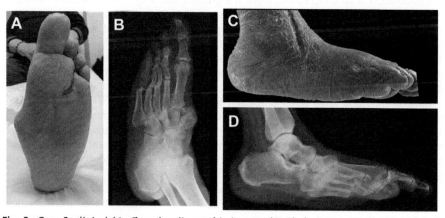

Fig. 9. *Case 2:* clinical (*A, C*) and radiographic images (*B, D*) during postoperative period, respectively, showing the progressive healing of the main plantar lesion and the DMOs performed on second to fifth MBs.

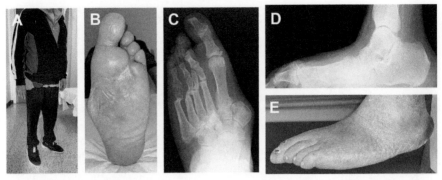

Fig. 10. *Case 2:* clinical and radiographic images at 10-month follow-up showing the patient standing and able to walk (*A*), complete healing of ulcers and their maintenance over time (*B–E*), and bone union (partial only for second MB) after the DMOs (*C, D*).

- *Nonhealing wound (23.8%) and bone necrosis (4.8%)*

Their rates are reported only by Tamir and colleagues[41]

- *Transfer lesions (9.1%-26.5%).*

These lesions are usually described under the heads of adjacent metatarsals,[26,39–42] as they occur when a correct metatarsal parabola is not re-established in the forefoot.[37] This is probably due to the resumption of patients' normal walking and incorrect overloading of the lateral MBs.

- *Ulcer recurrence (7.2%)*

The recurrence rate is higher in the first studies from the 90s,[42] whereas drastically decreases in later years.[26]

DISCUSSION

Although there has been a remarkable increase in knowledge on DFU healing mechanisms in recent years,[57] deficiencies in clinical DF ulceration management remain. As the population of DPs increases, there is a growing need for chronic wound management, and further research is needed to learn how to accelerate DFU healing and improve the quality of life for DPs. CPDFUs still represent the most severe and devastating complication in neuropathic DPs, representing a medical and surgical challenge in terms of treatment and a protracted process with high recurrence rates. Furthermore, the DPs who already have a DFU have a 2-year risk of 50.5% for another ulcer and 36.3% for amputation.[58]

Several methods have been proposed to treat plantar DFUs,[32–35] whose fundamental goal is to relieve the pressure, because "*the wound never heals until the pressure is off-loaded.*"[24] Among these, there are both conservative and operative solutions,[59] including bodyweight reduction, total contact casts,[60] removable walking boots, corrective shoes with a customized insole,[61] and even surgical correction, such as MH resection and ray amputation.[31–33,62]

However, in accordance with other authors,[63] we believe that total contact casts should no longer be used. It is our opinion that because of cast-related inconvenience and complications (difficult continuous ulcer monitoring, further skin lesions due to plaster in which fragmentation of the plaster causes ulcer contamination), many patients will not comply with the minimum 6 weeks of cast treatment before requesting to crossover to surgery, preferring more comfortable offloading methods such as a removable walking boot or a healing shoe. This is even more likely because patients now know about the new option of MIS.

Currently, intelligent socks and insoles are the main available wearable devices that show promising outcomes in the prevention of CPDFU.[64] There are smart socks, an optical fiber-based smart textile that allows the measurement of plantar foot temperature, and insole devices that monitor plantar pressure through specific sensors.[65] Recently, a proof-of-concept study conducted in the UK demonstrated that CPDFU recurrence can be significantly reduced by 71% compared with the standard of care by providing timely feedback on foot pressures to individuals through smart insoles.[66]

Moreover, a recent study shows that the incidence of first DFU, but not recurrent ulceration, is reduced in association with improvements in diabetes foot care. This is because prevention of DF ulceration has been difficult to achieve without a new balanced forefoot arch. Peripheral vascular disease, failure of ulcer healing, and age were associated with reduced survival, which after DFU has been historically poor.[67]

Hence, surgical treatment is indicated only after failure of 6-month conservative management. Several reports have shown the more traditional surgical procedures (MH resection, MB osteotomy and exostectomy, and arthrodesis) and tendon balancing (Achilles' tendon lengthening, gastrocnemius recession, and/or plantar fascia release) can achieve good to excellent results on DFU healing, regardless of their grade of severity and dimensions.[6,7,20] However, open surgical bone procedures are often correlated with high complication rates, such as ulcer recurrence or postoperative infection, whereas tendon balancing presents risks of tendon overlengthening, rupture, and plantar flexion weakness.[32,56,68] For these reasons, a conservative surgery preserving a toe, an MB, or a ray would be less traumatic and more acceptable by DPs, when feasible.[69]

In this context, MIS has been advised as an effective intervention,[35] becoming more popular because of its lower complication rates.[38] Diverse minimally invasive and percutaneous osteotomies, at different levels of the distal MBs, generally by a dorsal approach and without MB resection or internal fixation, have been proposed. These include osteoclasis, a V-shaped cut, a Gauthier osteotomy, or oblique cuts such as in a Weil osteotomy or its variants.[42,63] Their main common goals are as follows: *(1) the plantar DFUs healing by reducing the local pressure; and (2) the prevention of ulcer recurrence, transfer lesions, and local infections.*[37]

Owing to the preserved soft tissue covering and its characteristic stiffness in DF, the primary stability of these osteotomies is so high that successive osteosynthesis not only is unnecessary, but it would actually be harmful in preventing the dorsal elevation of the MB bone with respect to the ulcer level. In fact, the patient is asked to walk on the operated DF in the immediate postoperative period to elevate the MH dorsally and to release the plantar pressure.[69]

Furthermore, as DMOs do not require internal fixation, neither temporary (if not exceptionally using K-wires), the risk of infection of the metal implants is excluded, as well as the associated risk of osteomyelitis.[37,38] In DF, the main risk factors for developing osteomyelitis are the following: *(1) wounds that extend to bones or joints; and (2) previous history of a wound before enrollment, and recurrent or multiple wounds.* Most experts considered that the standard treatment of DF osteomyelitis should be the surgical removal of as much infected bone as possible while preserving foot function.[70,71] However, such surgical treatment modifies the shape and biomechanics of the foot and may predispose the patient to reulceration, which may be complicated again by bone infection and require a further amputation.

On the contrary, MIS by DMO completely changes the traditional surgical approach to CPFUs with osteomyelitis, preserving the infected MB such as the MH when possible. For this reason, we disagree with the view of previous articles supporting procedures that remove bone prominences and eliminate areas of high pressure in the foot but do not resolve the clinical and biomechanical problems because future consequences, such as transfer lesions or ulcer recurrences, are unavoidable without balancing the plantar pressures of the forefoot[24,38]

Supported by a systematic review with meta-analysis and metaregressions recently published[24] and personal clinical experience,[37,38] we strongly believe that DMOs can be a valid alternative treatment method also for CPDFUs with chronic infection, DFUs penetrating deep structures (IIIB, UTDWC[46,47]), and ulcers with osteomyelitis of the MBs or the P1. As the CPDFU represents the main access door for the bacteria causing foot osteomyelitis, resolving the first also promotes the healing of the second, avoiding long-term antibiotic therapy which causes progressive MB damage in DPs.[72]

The systematic review by the International Working Group on the Diabetic Foot states that "*no definitive statements can yet be made regarding the efficacy and safety of surgical interventions to heal DFUs or to prevent their recurrence, because of the limited number of RCTs.*"[62] We agree that MIS for CPDFUs by DMOs is a poorly investigated topic,[62] in contrast to the several traditional surgical techniques explored in the literature.[31–33,62] For this reason, there is a need for randomized controlled trials and prospective, longitudinal research studies, recruiting an adequate number of participants and investigating the combination of foot-loading factors, good glycaemic control, and their interaction on CPDFU healing. Certainly, higher quality evidence will better support and promote the use of DMOs as a treatment option for achieving and maintaining CPDFU healing in neuropathic DPs.

However, more recent systematic reviews[24,73] and previous several clinical series have shown successful outcomes for different offloading surgical procedures,[40,42,74,75] as have other clinicians with other procedures.[76] Evidence of clinical results has been reported, such as improvement and in most cases healing of the DFU and disappearance of the callosities that had developed at sites of pressure, within 2 to 3 weeks. Often, to achieve good outcomes, the DMOs are performed with 2 main associated procedures: (1) *percutaneous flexor tenotomy and phalanx osteotomies for tip of toe ulcers*[77,78] (in the same way as described previously by our protocol for additional procedures); and (2) *a modified Keller resection arthroplasty of the first MPJ for ulcers under the hallux*[79] (to this we prefer a modified Reverdin-Isham percutaneous osteotomy, performed a bit proximal to the I-MT neck).

Finally, previous DFU constitutes the highest risk for subsequent foot ulceration in diabetes,[27,80–83] and effective foot protection to reduce the number of reulceration is challenging.[84] For these reasons, we believe that the best approach to CPDFUs remains multidisciplinary, with a team that should include endocrinologists, podiatrists, wound care nurses, as well as vascular, general, and orthopedic surgeons, and infectious disease specialists. For CPDFU management, referral to a DF care clinic is also advised, not only for the most appropriate indication of treatment,[37] but also for first ulcer prevention with improved foot care services. It has been shown that adequate medical attendance of DF care services is necessary to prevent the first foot ulceration, and intensive diabetes counseling not only younger patients with DFUs can be useful.[67]

SUMMARY

In more than 30 years of scientific literature (1986–2021),[24] the few published studies on the management of CPDFUs by DMOs showed satisfactory short- to medium-term clinical and radiographic results. Although the reports systematically analyzed were all case series (level IV),[24] their data suggest that the DMOs, performed at different levels of the distal MBs, with very few contraindications (severe ischemia, gangrene, extensive soft tissue infection, and cellulitis) and low incidence of complications (excluding swelling), are an effective surgical treatment option for achieving rapid healing of CPDFUs (within 2 months) and preventing their recurrence after balancing of pressures in the forefeet of both type-1 and type-2 DPs.

DISCLOSURE

The authors have nothing to disclose.

CLINICS CARE POINTS

- At the first evaluation of a diabetic patient with CPDFU, classify the lesion according to the University of Texas wound classification system and ask for weight-bearing radiographs of the affected foot to identify the metatarsal bone/bones responsible for the ulceration.
- Plan medications and superficial debridement during the next visits, suggesting 6 weeks of off-loading orthotic treatment using a removable walking boot or corrective shoes with a customized insole. Avoid immediate surgery in the meantime.
- As an orthopedic surgeon, consider evaluating general comorbidities of the patient and his/her clinical progression with a multidisciplinary team (endocrinologists, podiatrists, wound care nurses, vascular and general surgeons, and infectious disease specialists). Avoid handling the patient alone.
- Conservative treatment rarely fails completely; more frequently it involves a reduction of the ulcer. The ideal time for minimally invasive surgery is when the dimensions of the ulcer have been stable for a couple of weeks. Avoid protracted nonoperative treatment for more than 6 weeks (except for extreme cases); this could lead to chronic lesions, infections, and osteomyelitis.
- Plan DMOs not only according to clinical aspects but also using Maestro radiographic criteria to avoid recurrences. Use proper surgical equipment and follow the procedure and postoperative protocol as described. Avoid treating additional lesions and deformities with a single operation; this could lead to ischemia of the toes and forefoot in the days following the operation.

DISCLOSURE

The authors have nothing to disclose.

REFERENCES

1. Abbott CA, Carrington AL, Ashe H, et al. The north-west diabetes foot care study: incidence of, and risk factors for, new diabetic foot ulceration in a community-based patient cohort. Diabet Med 2002;19(5):377–84.
2. Boyko EJ, Ahroni JH, Cohen V, et al. Prediction of diabetic foot ulcer occurrence using commonly available clinical information: the Seattle Diabetic Foot Study. Diabetes care 2006;29(6):1202–7.
3. Margolis DJ, Malay DS, Hoffstad OJ, et al. Incidence of diabetic foot ulcer and lower extremity amputation among Medicare beneficiaries, 2006 to 2008: Data Points# 2. 2011, In: Data Points Publication Series [Internet], Rockville (MD): Agency for Healthcare Research and Quality (US).

4. Zhang P, Lu J, Jing Y, et al. Global epidemiology of diabetic foot ulceration: a systematic review and meta-analysis (†). Ann Med 2017;49(2):106–16.
5. Prompers L, Huijberts M, Apelqvist J, et al. High prevalence of ischaemia, infection and serious comorbidity in patients with diabetic foot disease in Europe. Baseline results from the Eurodiale study. Diabetologia 2007;50(1):18–25.
6. Batista F, Magalhaes AA, Nery C, et al. Minimally invasive surgery for diabetic plantar foot ulcerations. Diabet Foot Ankle 2011;2(1):10358.
7. Ahmad J. The diabetic foot. Diabetes Metab Syndr 2016;10(1):48–60.
8. Muduli IC, Ansar PP, Panda C, et al. Diabetic foot ulcer complications and its management-a medical college-based descriptive study in odisha, an Eastern State of India. Indian J Surg 2015;77(Suppl 2):270–4.
9. Lipsky BA, Berendt AR, Cornia PB, et al. 2012 Infectious Diseases Society of America clinical practice guideline for the diagnosis and treatment of diabetic foot infections. Clin Infect Dis 2012;54(12):e132–73.
10. Vadiveloo T, Jeffcoate W, Donnan PT, et al. Amputation-free survival in 17,353 people at high risk for foot ulceration in diabetes: a national observational study. Diabetologia 2018;61(12):2590–7.
11. Walsh JW, Hoffstad OJ, Sullivan MO, et al. Association of diabetic foot ulcer and death in a population-based cohort from the United Kingdom. Diabetic Med 2016;33(11):1493–8.
12. Hex N, Bartlett C, Wright D, et al. Estimating the current and future costs of Type 1 and Type 2 diabetes in the UK, including direct health costs and indirect societal and productivity costs. Diabetic Med 2012;29(7):855–62.
13. Monteiro-Soares M, Boyko EJ, Ribeiro J, et al. Predictive factors for diabetic foot ulceration: a systematic review. Diabetes Metab Res Rev 2012;28(7):574–600.
14. Cowley MS, Boyko EJ, Shofer JB, et al. Foot ulcer risk and location in relation to prospective clinical assessment of foot shape and mobility among persons with diabetes. Diabetes Res Clin Pract 2008;82(2):226–32.
15. Helal B. Metatarsal osteotomy for metatarsalgia. J Bone Joint Surg Br 1975;57(2):187–92.
16. Lavery LA, Lavery DC, Quebedeax-Farnham TL. Increased foot pressures after great toe amputation in diabetes. Diabetes Care 1995;18(11):1460–2.
17. Lázaro-Martínez JL, Aragón-Sánchez FJ, Beneit-Montesinos JV, et al. Foot biomechanics in patients with diabetes mellitus: doubts regarding the relationship between neuropathy, foot motion, and deformities. J Am Podiatr Med Assoc 2011;101(3):208–14.
18. Tamir E, Vigler M, Avisar E, et al. Percutaneous tenotomy for the treatment of diabetic toe ulcers. Foot Ankle Int 2014;35(1):38–43.
19. Todros S, Biz C, Ruggieri P, et al. Experimental analysis of plantar fascia mechanical properties in subjects with foot pathologies. Appl Sci 2021;11(4):1517.
20. Armstrong DG, Boulton AJM, Bus SA. Diabetic foot ulcers and their recurrence. N Engl J Med 2017;376(24):2367–75.
21. Hinchliffe RJ, Brownrigg JR, Andros G, et al. Effectiveness of revascularization of the ulcerated foot in patients with diabetes and peripheral artery disease: a systematic review. Diabetes Metab Res Rev 2016;32(Suppl 1):136–44.
22. Bus SA, Armstrong DG, van Deursen RW, et al. IWGDF guidance on footwear and offloading interventions to prevent and heal foot ulcers in patients with diabetes. Diabetes Metab Res Rev 2016;32(Suppl 1):25–36.
23. Fibreglass total contact casting, removable cast walkers, and irremovable cast walkers to treat diabetic neuropathic foot ulcers: a health technology assessment. Ont Health Technol Assess Ser 2017;17(12):1–124.

24. Biz C, Belluzzi E, Crimì A, et al. Minimally invasive metatarsal osteotomies (Mimos) for the treatment of plantar diabetic forefoot ulcers (pdfus): A systematic review and meta-analysis with meta-regressions. Appl Sci (Switzerland) 2021; 11(20):1–21.

25. Lavery LA, Higgins KR, La Fontaine J, et al. Randomised clinical trial to compare total contact casts, healing sandals and a shear-reducing removable boot to heal diabetic foot ulcers. Int Wound J 2015;12(6):710–5.

26. Tamir E, Tamar M, Ayalon M, et al. Effect of mini-invasive floating metatarsal osteotomy on plantar pressure in patients with diabetic plantar metatarsal head ulcers. Foot Ankle Int 2021;42(5):536–43.

27. Apelqvist J, Larsson J, Agardh CD. Long-term prognosis for diabetic patients with foot ulcers. J Intern Med 1993;233(6):485–91.

28. Dubský M, Jirkovská A, Bem R, et al. Risk factors for recurrence of diabetic foot ulcers: prospective follow-up analysis in the Eurodiale subgroup. Int Wound J 2013;10(5):555–61.

29. Biz C, Fosser M, Dalmau-Pastor M, et al. Functional and radiographic outcomes of hallux valgus correction by mini-invasive surgery with Reverdin-Isham and Akin percutaneous osteotomies: a longitudinal prospective study with a 48-month follow-up. J Orthop Surg Res 2016;11(1):157.

30. Bauer T, de Lavigne C, Biau D, et al. Percutaneous hallux valgus surgery: a prospective multicenter study of 189 cases. Orthop Clin North Am 2009;40(4): 505–14, ix.

31. Dayer R, Assal M. Chronic diabetic ulcers under the first metatarsal head treated by staged tendon balancing: a prospective cohort study. J Bone Joint Surg Br Volume 2009;91(4):487–93.

32. Cychosz CC, Phisitkul P, Belatti DA, et al. Preventive and therapeutic strategies for diabetic foot ulcers. Foot Ankle Int 2015;37(3):334–43.

33. Willrich A, Angirasa AK, Sage RA. Percutaneous tendo Achillis lengthening to promote healing of diabetic plantar foot ulceration. J Am Podiatric Med Assoc 2005;95(3):281–4.

34. Dallimore SM, Kaminski MR. Tendon lengthening and fascia release for healing and preventing diabetic foot ulcers: a systematic review and meta-analysis. J Foot Ankle Res 2015;8:33.

35. La Fontaine J, Lavery LA, Hunt NA, et al. The role of surgical off-loading to prevent recurrent ulcerations. Int J Low Extrem Wounds 2014;13(4):320–34.

36. Hamilton GA, Ford LA, Perez H, et al. Salvage of the neuropathic foot by using bone resection and tendon balancing: a retrospective review of 10 patients. J Foot Ankle Surg 2005;44(1):37–43.

37. Biz C, Ruggieri P. Minimally Invasive Surgery: Osteotomies for Diabetic Foot Disease. Foot Ankle Clin 2020;25(3):441–60.

38. Biz C, Gastaldo S, Dalmau-Pastor M, et al. Minimally invasive distal metatarsal diaphyseal osteotomy (DMDO) for chronic plantar diabetic foot ulcers. Foot Ankle Int 2018;39(1):83–92.

39. Chiu WK, Yang TF, Wang HJ, et al. Assessment of outcomes of a metatarsal bone ostectomy for chronic plantar ulcers: a preliminary study. Ann Plast Surg 2020; 84(1S Suppl 1):s112–5.

40. Tamir E, Finestone AS, Avisar E, et al. Mini-Invasive floating metatarsal osteotomy for resistant or recurrent neuropathic plantar metatarsal head ulcers. J Orthopaedic Surg Res 2016;11(1):78.

41. Tamir E, Smorgick Y, Ron GZ, et al. Mini invasive floating metatarsal osteotomy for diabetic foot ulcers under the first metatarsal head: a case series. Int J Lower Extremity Wounds 2020;1–6.

42. Tillo TH, Giurini JM, Habershaw GM, et al. Review of metatarsal osteotomies for the treatment of neuropathic ulcerations. J Am Podiatric Med Assoc 1990;80(4): 211–7.

43. Wray C. The Helal osteotomy in a diabetic patient. Pract Diabetes Int 1986; 3(3):156.

44. Finestone AS, Tamir E, Ron G, et al. Surgical offloading procedures for diabetic foot ulcers compared to best non-surgical treatment: a study protocol for a randomized controlled trial. J Foot Ankle Res 2018;11(6):1–9.

45. Biz C, Corradin M, Kuete Kanah WT, et al. Medium-long-Term clinical and radiographic outcomes of minimally invasive Distal Metatarsal Metaphyseal Osteotomy (DMMO) for central primary metatarsalgia: do maestro criteria have a predictive value in the preoperative planning for this percutaneous technique? Biomed Res Int 2018;2018:1947024.

46. Redfern DJ, Vernois J. Percutaneous surgery for metatarsalgia and the lesser toes. Foot Ankle Clin 2016;21(3):527–50.

47. Lavery LA, Armstrong DG, Harkless LB. Classification of diabetic foot wounds. J Foot Ankle Surg 1996;35(6):528–31.

48. Oyibo SO, Jude EB, Tarawneh I, et al. A comparison of two diabetic foot ulcer classification systems: the Wagner and the University of Texas wound classification systems. Diabetes Care 2001;24(1):84–8.

49. Coughlin M, Mann R, Saltzman C. Surgery of the foot and ankle. Philadelphia: Mosby; 2007. p. 1289.

50. Maestro M, Besse J-L, Ragusa M, et al. Forefoot morphotype study and planning method for forefoot osteotomy. Foot Ankle Clin 2003;8(4):695–710.

51. Biz C, de Iudicibus G, Belluzzi E, et al. Prevalence of chronic pain syndrome in patients who have undergone hallux valgus percutaneous surgery: a comparison of sciatic-femoral and ankle regional ultrasound-guided nerve blocks. BMC Musculoskelet Disord 2021;22(1):1043.

52. Muñoz-García N, Tomé-Bermejo F, Herrera-Molpeceres J. Pseudoarthrosis after distal percutaneous osteotomy of lower distal radii. Revista Española de Cirugía Ortopédica y Traumatología (English Edition) 2011;55(1):31–4.

53. Kim PJ, Steinberg JS. Wound care: biofilm and its impact on the latest treatment modalities for ulcerations of the diabetic foot. Semin Vasc Surg 2012;25(2):70–4.

54. Lebrun E, Tomic-Canic M, Kirsner RS. The role of surgical debridement in healing of diabetic foot ulcers. Wound Repair Regen 2010;18(5):433–8.

55. Biz C, Corradin M, Petretta I, et al. Endolog technique for correction of hallux valgus: a prospective study of 30 patients with 4-year follow-up. J Orthop Surg Res 2015;10:102.

56. Biz C, Crimì A, Fantoni I, et al. Functional and radiographic outcomes of Minimally invasive Intramedullary Nail Device (MIIND) for moderate to severe hallux valgus. Foot Ankle Int 2021;42(4):409–24.

57. Fleischli JE, Anderson RB, Davis WH. Dorsiflexion metatarsal osteotomy for treatment of recalcitrant diabetic neuropathic ulcers. Foot Ankle Int 1999;20(2):80–5.

58. Burgess JL, Wyant WA, Abdo Abujamra B, et al. Diabetic wound-healing science. Medicina 2021;57(10):1072.

59. Lavery LA, Peters EJ, Williams JR, et al. Reevaluating the way we classify the diabetic foot: restructuring the diabetic foot risk classification system of the International Working Group on the Diabetic Foot. Diabetes Care 2008;31(1):154–6.

60. Singh N, Armstrong DG, Lipsky BA. Preventing foot ulcers in patients with diabetes. JAMA 2005;293(2):217–28.
61. Wukich DK, Motko J. Safety of total contact casting in high-risk patients with neuropathic foot ulcers. Foot Ankle Int 2004;25(8):556–60.
62. Rizzo L, Tedeschi A, Fallani E, et al. Custom-made orthesis and shoes in a structured follow-up program reduces the incidence of neuropathic ulcers in high-risk diabetic foot patients. Int J Lower Extrem Wounds 2012;11(1):59–64.
63. Yammine K, Assi C. Surgical offloading techniques should be used more often and earlier in treating forefoot diabetic ulcers: an evidence-based review. Int J Lower Extrem Wounds 2019. 1534734619888361.
64. Najafi B, Reeves ND, Armstrong DG. Leveraging smart technologies to improve the management of diabetic foot ulcers and extend ulcer-free days in remission. Diabetes Metab Res Rev 2020;36(Suppl 1):e3239.
65. Orlando G, Prior Y, Reeves ND, et al. Patient and provider perspective of smart wearable technology in diabetic foot ulcer prevention: a systematic review. Medicina (Kaunas) 2021;57(12):1359.
66. Abbott CA, Chatwin KE, Foden P, et al. Innovative intelligent insole system reduces diabetic foot ulcer recurrence at plantar sites: a prospective, randomised, proof-of-concept study. Lancet Digital Health 2019;1(6):e308–18.
67. Paisey RB, Abbott A, Paisey CF, et al. Diabetic foot ulcer incidence and survival with improved diabetic foot services: an 18-year study. Diabetic Med 2019; 36(11):1424–30.
68. Lin SS, Lee TH, Wapner KL. Plantar forefoot ulceration with equinus deformity of the ankle in diabetic patients: the effect of tendo-Achilles lengthening and total contact casting. Orthopedics 1996;19(5):465–75.
69. Yammine K, Assi C. Conservative surgical options for the treatment of forefoot diabetic ulcers and osteomyelitis: an evidence-based review and a decision-making tool. JBJS Rev 2020;8(6):e0162.
70. Jeffcoate WJ, Lipsky BA, Berendt AR, et al. Unresolved issues in the management of ulcers of the foot in diabetes. Diabetic Med 2008;25(12):1380–9.
71. Lipsky BA, Uçkay İ. Treating diabetic foot osteomyelitis: a practical state-of-the-art update. Medicina 2021;57(4):339.
72. Aragón-Sánchez J, Lázaro-Martínez JL, Alvaro-Afonso FJ, et al. Conservative surgery of diabetic forefoot osteomyelitis: how can I operate on this patient without amputation? Int J Lower Extremity Wounds 2014;14(2):108–31.
73. Yammine K, Nahed M, Assi C. Metatarsal Osteotomies for treating neuropathic diabetic foot ulcers: a meta-analysis. Foot Ankle Spec 2019;12(6):555–62.
74. Elraiyah T, Prutsky G, Domecq JP, et al. A systematic review and meta-analysis of off-loading methods for diabetic foot ulcers. J Vasc Surg 2016;63(2 Suppl): 59S–68S, e51-52.
75. Götz J, Lange M, Dullien S, et al. Off-loading strategies in diabetic foot syndrome-evaluation of different devices. Int Orthop 2017;41(2):239–46.
76. Laffenêtre O, Perera A. Distal minimally invasive metatarsal Osteotomy ("DMMO" Procedure). Foot Ankle Clin 2019;24(4):615–25.
77. Schepers T, Berendsen HA, Oei IH, et al. Functional outcome and patient satisfaction after flexor tenotomy for plantar ulcers of the toes. J Foot Ankle Surg 2010;49(2):119–22.
78. Tamir E, Vigler M, Avisar E, et al. Percutaneous tenotomy for the treatment of diabetic toe ulcers. Foot Ankle Int 2013;35(1):38–43.
79. Tamir E, Tamir J, Beer Y, et al. Resection arthroplasty for resistant ulcers underlying the hallux in insensate diabetics. Foot Ankle Int 2015;36(8):969–75.

80. Crawford F, Cezard G, Chappell FM. The development and validation of a multivariable prognostic model to predict foot ulceration in diabetes using a systematic review and individual patient data meta-analyses. Diabetic Med 2018;35(11): 1480–93.
81. Lincoln NB, Radford KA, Game FL, et al. Education for secondary prevention of foot ulcers in people with diabetes: a randomised controlled trial. Diabetologia 2008;51(11):1954–61.
82. Örneholm H, Apelqvist J, Larsson J, et al. Recurrent and other new foot ulcers after healed plantar forefoot diabetic ulcer. Wound Repair Regen 2017;25(2): 309–15.
83. Armstrong DG, Bharara M, White M, et al. The impact and outcomes of establishing an integrated interdisciplinary surgical team to care for the diabetic foot. Diabetes Metab Res Rev 2012;28(6):514–8.
84. Reiber GE, Smith DG, Wallace C, et al. Effect of therapeutic footwear on foot reulceration in patients with diabetes: a randomized controlled trial. JAMA 2002; 287(19):2552–8.

NEMISIS: Neuropathic Minimally Invasive Surgeries. Charcot Midfoot Reconstruction, Surgical Technique, Pearls and Pitfalls

Roslyn Miller, FRCS Tr&Orth, MBChB, BscMed Sci[a,b,c]

KEYWORDS

- Minimally invasive surgery • Percutaneous • Charcot • Midfoot deformity
- Rocker bottom • Diabetic foot disease

KEY POINTS

- Early surgical intervention decreases reulceration and amputation rates, which in turn decrease morbidity and mortality.
- Percutaneous Achilles tendon lengthening and exostectomy can be performed in stable rocker-bottom deformity.
- Combining the surgical techniques of minimally invasive surgery and the superconstruct with advances in implant technology facilitates large deformity correction through percutaneous incisions.
- In the management of diabetic foot disease, the role of the orthopedic surgeon within the multidisciplinary team is fundamental to correct deformity and abnormal biomechanics.
- Neuropathic minimally invasive surgeries facilitate day surgery procedures with regional anesthesia, which are beneficial to the recovery of planned services after the coronavirus disease 2019 pandemic.

INTRODUCTION

The number of patients with diabetes continues to increase.[1,2] So too do the risks associated with diabetic foot disease to the patient. Resources and financial burden on health care systems before the coronavirus disease 2019 pandemic had already increased. Significant progress had been made toward decreasing morbidity and mortality principally by the collaborative working of the multidisciplinary diabetic foot team.[1,3–12]

[a] NHS Lanarkshire Universities Hospitals, Lanarkshire, Scotland, UK; [b] Glasgow Caledonian University, Glasgow, Scotland, UK; [c] Department of Orthopaedics, Foot and Ankle Service Lead, Hairmyres University Hospital, 218 Eaglesham Road, East Kilbride, Glasgow G75 8RG, UK
E-mail address: rosmiller@doctors.org.uk
Twitter: @footdoctoruk (R.M.)

Foot Ankle Clin N Am 27 (2022) 567–581
https://doi.org/10.1016/j.fcl.2022.05.001
1083-7515/22/Crown Copyright © 2022 Published by Elsevier Inc. All rights reserved.

foot.theclinics.com

It is recognized that patients who develop Charcot and foot deformity have their quality of life severely negatively impacted by the acquired deformity.[13] This patient group has substantial improvement in patient-reported outcomes relating to their quality of life after surgery.[14] Early intervention for patients at risk of ulceration results in significant decrease in amputation rates.[3,4,12,15] This practice in turn has a major impact on decreasing the financial burden of diabetic foot disease on health care systems.[11,16,17]

The coronavirus disease 2019 pandemic has had a significant impact on the management of these patients. During the initial 3-month lock-down from March to June 2020, the decrease in mobility, coupled with family members being at home anecdotally saw a decrease in active ulceration in the UK.

The well-established conservative management by diabetic podiatrists and orthotists of diabetic ulcers with meticulous surgical debridement, wound management, and off-loading with total contact casting facilitated the healing and maintenance of ulcers. The imperative to protect the capacity of the National Heath Service meant that patients who could be managed conservatively were. However, it is well-established that there is a significant reulceration rate that significantly increases mortality at 5 years. Collection of routine data regarding ulceration rates in Scotland has been limited during 2020 to 2022, but anecdotally the amputation rates have begun to increase again, which patients having a greater burden of medical comorbidities. There has also been a significant increase in the number of patients presenting with active Charcot arthropathy unable to access reconstructive surgery.

Correction of the abnormal biomechanics in patients with diabetic foot disease secondary to neuropathy promotes ulcer healing and decreases reulceration rates. With advances in surgical techniques and technology over the last few decades has come the evolution of the subspecialist orthopedic foot and ankle surgeon, declaring a real interest in the surgical management and reconstruction of these complex cases.[18]

Fundamental to the recovery of planned services is the optimization of treatment strategies to minimize hospital attendances owing to repeated problems such as recurrent ulceration from abnormal peak pressures because of deformity secondary to Charcot neuroarthropathy. These major reconstructions offer patients not only an increase in life expectancy secondary to a decrease in reulceration rates, but an improved quality of life as a result of fewer regular visits to the hospital and the ability to get into more "normal" custom footwear.[14]

Surgical reconstruction of a deformity of the foot and ankle is technically challenging. Modern fixation techniques using the principles of superconstructs and extended arthrodesis have resulted in a paradigm shift in the management of complex Charcot neuroarthropathy.[19] As industry has embraced the development of Charcot-specific reconstruction systems, the surgeon now has the tools to address complex limb salvage in Charcot neuroarthropathy.[19] The advances in surgical techniques of minimally invasive surgery, coupled with the development of new surgical implants facilitated a transition to earlier surgical intervention in these patients with the aim now of preventing significant, difficult-to-manage deformities.

MIDFOOT CHARCOT

Patients with midfoot Charcot neuroarthropathy are at risk of developing a rocker bottom deformity. The gradual and progressive destruction of the architecture of the midfoot arch increases the risk of ulceration and osteomyelitis increases the risk of ulceration.[8] The medial column is typically first affected.[20] The deformity may remain static at the medial column or may progress over time to the lateral column.

Sensorimotor and autonomic neuropathy results in progressive tightness of the gastric soleus muscle complex secondary to changes in collagen fibers and owing to glycosylation. This process causes and equinus deformity of the ankle and talus, with or without cuneiforms. Opposing forces are from the tibialis anterior and posterior muscles distally.[8,21,22] Failure of the plantar osseous–ligamentous structures result in a midfoot break. The increased peak plantar pressures in the forefoot and midfoot result in a typical rocker bottom with subsequent ulceration.

CLASSIFICATION

The classification systems of Eichenholz and Brodsky are based on the clinical, anatomic, and radiological location of the disease.[23,24] Tiruveedhula and colleague's[25] classification combines the clinical features and radiographic parameters with the anatomic location of the disease to determine which patients would benefit from percutaneous tendo-Achilles lengthening and total contact casting. Sammarco and Conti's midfoot classification[26] helps to determine which midfoot pattern may benefit from the superconstruct fixation method.

BENEFITS OF NEUROPATHIC MINIMALLY INVASIVE SURGERIES

There are certain circumstances where neuropathic minimally invasive surgery (NEMISIS) performed via percutaneous incisions under fluoroscopic guidance have significant advantages. Historically, management of the acute phase of Charcot neuroarthropathy has been total contact casting. NEMISIS combined with implants specifically designed for Charcot reconstruction mean early surgical intervention in the acute phase to prevent deformity is now possible. NEMISIS also affords the surgeon the potential to correct deformity and decrease the ulceration risk when conditions are unable to be optimized further. In patients who are noncompliant or who have persistently elevated hemoglobin A1c levels, unreconstructed vascular disease, and/or have significant comorbidities,[27] NEMISIS provides the surgeon with a technique to minimize, although not fully eliminate, the perioperative and postoperative risks. This procedure, coupled with careful preoperative optimization of the patients' comorbidities and the use of regional anesthesia, helps to mitigate risk for this patient group as much as is possible.

There is an absolute indication for surgery in the acute phase of midfoot Charcot neuroarthropathy, when there is early radiological evidence of extrusion of the navicular or medial cuneiform.[27] Surgery at this stage, during the evolution of the arthropathy, allows stabilization of the medial column, preventing deformity and the subsequent skin necrosis that often results. In the latter stages of Charcot neuroarthropathy, where the bone has coalesced and reconstituted, the deformity is stable. However, the deformity produces high pressure areas that result in skin necrosis and ulcer formation. In this situation, an exostectomy to remove the bony prominence will allow the redistribution of forces across the whole foot and decrease the risk of further ulceration.

Caution is required when performing an exostectomy. Surgery should only be performed when the foot is stable with fused midfoot joints. Exosteostectomy of the undersurface of the midfoot when the joints have not fused risks exacerbating the deformity.[27]

PATIENT SELECTION

The optimal patient for NEMISIS for Charcot neuroarthropathy has sufficient skin cover with no active ulceration and sufficient bone stock to facilitate reconstruction with intramedullary beams and bolts.[28]

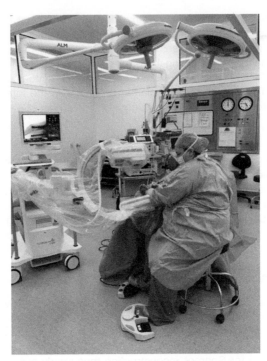

Fig. 1. Operating room setup–patient positioning and the mini-C arm.

PROCEDURE
Preoperative Prophylaxis

Five days of Nacetpin nasal cream and Hibiscrub is prescribed to reduce the risk of postoperative infection from meticillin-sensitive *Staphylococcus* aureus (MSSA).[2,29]

Admission and Anesthesia

The patient is admitted as an inpatient, and surgery is performed under general anesthesia with a popliteal block and intravenous antibiotics after bone biopsies (usually flucloxacillin and gentamicin, depending on previous sensitivities, allergies, and renal function).

Surgical setup

The patient is placed supine on the operating table with the feet off the end of the bed to allow for easy access of the mini-C arm. A bump under the ipsilateral hip brings the foot to neutral. The leg is usually prepared to the knee to allow for the possibility of external fixation application.

The operating table should be positioned in the theater with the feet centered under the operating lights, to ensure that there is sufficient space for the mini-C arm and equipment. The mini-C arm is used for intraoperative fluoroscopy, which should come in from the end of the bed, for maximum maneuverability. Calf tourniquet (if pulses present) is used (**Fig. 1**).

1. Achilles tendon and the equinus talus

The first stage in midfoot reconstruction is to assess for tightness in the Achilles tendon causing equinus of the talus and contributing to the midfoot break.

Percutaneous Achilles tendon lengthening or gastrocnemius recession provides adequate lengthening of the Achilles to allow the calcaneus to become plantigrade and correction of the alignment of the talus with the first metatarsal.[22,25]

2. The triplanar closing wedge

The medially based midfoot osteotomy is a multifaceted correction of the midfoot and forefoot which allows for correction mostly in the sagittal and transverse planes.[29,30] This biplanar osteotomy removes a triplanar closing wedge, **Fig. 2**, and is typically used in severe Charcot deformity involving multiple joints of the midfoot.[29,30]

There are 2 × 2 mm K-wires or Steinman pins inserted from medial to lateral under fluoroscopic guidance encompassing the apex of the deformity to act a cutting tract, **Fig. 3**.

A dorsal, medial, longitudinal, percutaneous stab incision is made with a Beaver blade along the medial column centrally located over the apex of the deformity, **Fig. 4**. A 2 × 20 mm and the 3 × 20 mm Shannon cutting burr is used to create the 2 osteotomies that form the wedge, **Fig. 5**. These osteotomies frequently need to be performed in 2 stages at the burrs may not reach the plantar aspect of the foot in a single pass. This is especially the case if there is significant dislocation of the midtarsal joints. A 3.1-mm wedge burr, **Fig. 6**, is used to 'mill' the bone and convert the bone into a bone paste.

When the osteotomies have been made correctly, with sufficient removal of bone, the forefoot should be fully mobile (**Fig. 7**) and allows for closure on the medial side with a plantar flexion force when the osteotomy is fixated.

If the full depth of bone is not completely removed, the medial column may not be able to be reduced in the correct alignment to restore Mearys' angle. Another reason that the reduction may not be achievable is if the lateral column is too stiff to allow abduction of the forefoot. A second lateral incision is often required to free the lateral column and essentially transect the midfoot to allow repositioning of the forefoot relative to the proximal midfoot in any plane.

3. Beams and bolts, the superconstruct and intermedullary foot fixation

Grant[31] first described the principle of the technique to reconstruct the midfoot following deformity caused by Charcot neuroarthropathy. The concept of the superconstruct (**Fig. 8**), which spans adjacent joints, was introduce by Sammarco.[32]

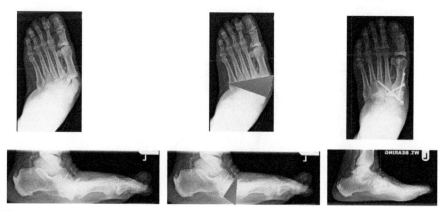

Fig. 2. Triplanar closing wedge osteotomy.

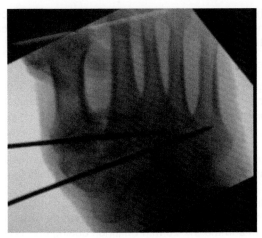

Fig. 3. A K-wire placement as the guide for an osteotomy.

There are 4 factors that define the superconstruct:

a. Fusion beyond the zone of injury to include unaffected joints to provided improve fixation.
b. Bone resection to shorten the extremity, allowing adequate reduction of the deformity without tension on the soft tissue envelope.
c. Using the strongest device that can be tolerated by the soft tissue envelope.
d. Applying the device in a position to maximizes mechanical function.

Lamm and colleagues[33] describe the benefits of intermedullary foot fixation for midfoot Charcot deformity correction as allowing:

a. Anatomic realignment
b. inimally invasive fixation technique
c. Formal multiple joint fusion
d. Adjacent joint fixation beyond the level of Charcot collapse
e. Rigid interosseus fixation
f. Preservation of foot length
g. Combined with external fixation if necessary.

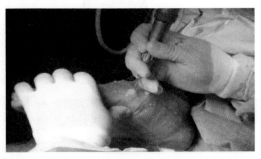

Fig. 4. Access for plantar medial exostectomy.

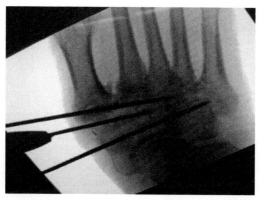

Fig. 5. The Shannon cutting burr.

4. The medial column

The decision as to whether fixation should be with an intermedullary superconstruct or not depends on the site of deformity and the degree of translation or dislocation of midfoot joints. Where the deformity is located at the tarsometatarsal joints, the first tarsometatarsal joint should be reduced and held with a screw placed percutaneously from the first metatarsal head to the medial cuneiform. Supplementary fixation of the first to second or first to third tarsometatarsal joints should then be sufficient[27] **(Fig. 9)**.

If there is severe fragmentation of the navicular bone with involvement of the perinavicular joints, then it is impossible to spare the talonavicular joint. Arthrodesis of the talonavicular joint with or without arthrodesis of the subtalar joint is then indicated.[32] Dorsal dislocation of the midfoot joints, whether at the tarsometatarsal, naviculocuneiform, or talonavicular joints, requires spanning of the medial column. This procedure can be performed either antegrade through the first metatarsal head or retrograde from the talus.[27,32–34]

5. The middle column

A single beam or bolt to the medial column is not usually sufficient fixation and a further 5 mm bolt should be placed into the second and or third metatarsal to cuneiform or talus. It is usually easier to fix the second metatarsal first, like principles of Lisfranc fixation, **Fig. 10**. If there is significant calcification of the Lisfranc ligament, this will need to be taken down with the 3-mm wedge burr to allow the reduction to take place.

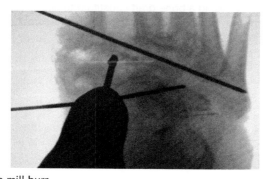

Fig. 6. The wedge mill burr.

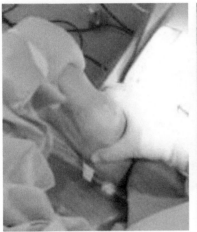
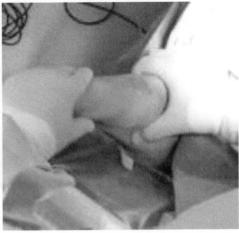

Fig. 7. Deformity correction.

6. The lateral column

If there is any involvement of the lateral column this should be fixated with 5-mm bolts going from the fourth and or fifth metatarsal to the cuboid or calcaneum (**Fig. 11**). The lateral column is very unstable and prone to recurrence of the rocker bottom deformity.

CLINICS CARE POINTS

- Ensure the patient is placed operating table with the feet off the end of the bed, to allow for easy access of the mini-C arm.
- Percutaneous Achilles tendon lengthening or gastrocnemius recession provides adequate lengthening of the Achilles tendon allow the calcaneus to become plantigrade.
- Place the initial percutaneous incision at the apex of the deformity.
- Anticipate that additional approaches may be requires as the burr may not reach the full depth of the deformity.
- Ensure the osteotomy reached lateral aspect of the midfoot to allow for full correction of the midfoot position.
- If there is any history of a previous infected ulcer, remove all bone paste and wash out. Consider using a bone graft substitute to fill the void.
- Place guidewires to reduce and hold the second tarsometatarsal joint before placing a 7-mm beam to the first ray.

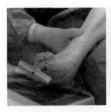
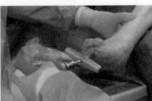

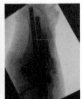

Fig. 8. The superconstruct.

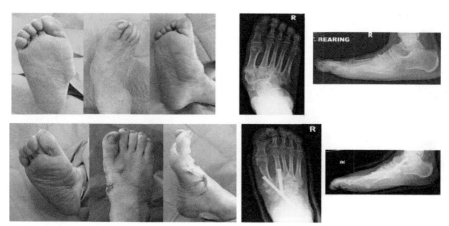

Fig. 9. Midfoot rocker bottom correction.

- Once the middle and medial columns have been reduced and held with beams and bolts, asses the lateral column. If any rocker bottom deformity present, place a beam from the fifth and/or fourth metatarsal to the calcaneus, crossing the cuboid.

POSTOPERATIVELY

The foot is placed into a below-knee backslab that extends beyond the toes. Care must be taken when applying the backslab that the ankle is dorsiflexed at the hindfoot and not at the forefoot, because this will encourage stress across the midfoot and potential to increase risk of hardware failure.

The patient is discharged the following day on oral antibiotics and nonweightbearing. They are then seen for a wound check at 3 and 7 days. At 1 week, they are then placed into a full plaster cast, extending beyond the toes, with an axial off-loader. The

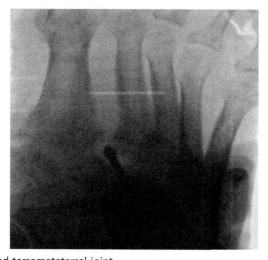

Fig. 10. The second tarsometatarsal joint.

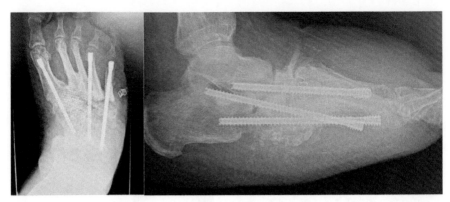

Fig. 11. The lateral column.

foot can become swollen in the early stages, with erythematous changes similar to a reactivation of charcot neuroarthropathy (CN). This is usually a result of extruded bone graft substitute can leak out of the incision. If this is the case the, patient should remain on oral antibiotics, with weekly checks undertaken until the foot shows clinical signs of stability.

Once the early signs of stability are evident (reduced swelling, temperature, and pain if the patient has any residual sensation) the limb is then placed into a moonboot with total contact insole, until custom footwear is available.

COMPLICATIONS
Arthrodesis and Nonunion

The goal of surgery is to achieve a stable plantigrade foot with a solid arthrodesis. However, it has been demonstrated that a robust fibrous nonunion can still facilitate transition to footwear without loss of correction and reulceration.[2,29,32,35,36] There may be some loss of correction secondary to nonunion, but this is not sufficient to create the high peak pressure associated with ulcer formation.

Migration and Hardware Failure

Two types of percutaneous fixation can be used. The midfoot or medial column bolt is a solid bolt with a threaded tip and head. There are a range of diameters of fixation with the 5.0-mm or 5.5-mm bolt commonly used for the middle and lateral columns.[19,37,38] A larger 6.5-mm bolt is used for the medial column. Reports of migration of medial the medial column bolt[34,39] can be mitigated against by using a thread beam instead of a short, shallow threaded bolt. Cannulated threaded beams allow of reduction and fixation of the medial column.[2,28,33,40] However, hardware failure is a recognized complication of beams and bolts (**Fig. 12**), as high as 60%, although the actual numbers of patients in the series are low.[28] A solid, stainless steel beam may be technically more challenging to place, but the increased stiffness owing to a higher Young's modulus of elasticity compared with titanium may prove advantageous with less of a risk of breakage.[33]

INFECTION AND AMPUTATION

The overall risk of complications after reconstructive surgery for Charcot neuroarthropathy is approximately 36%.[35] Reconstructive surgery in patients with Charcot neuroarthropathy carries a high risk of infection.[2,28,41,42] However,

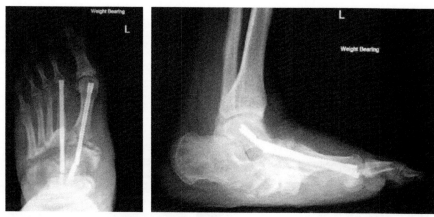

Fig. 12. Complications: Breakage of implants.

amputation rates remain low after reconstructive surgery at an average of 5.5%. Most reassuring is that 91% of patients return to ambulation after surgical reconstruction.[35]

The use of an injectable, antibiotic-loaded bone graft substitute into the void created by the resection of the wedge is used routinely by this author. This step ensures the local delivery of antibiotic directly to the surgical site. It also has the benefit of not placing an increased burden on the patients' renal function because the drug is not administered systemically. The patient is then able to be discharged home on a lower dose of oral antibiotics.

In this author's experience in cases where infection of the hardware has occurred, removal of the hardware, with washout and 6 weeks of antibiotics has resulted in resolution of the infection. Critically however, the corrected position has been maintained without recurrence of deformity (**Fig. 13**).

SINGLE- VERSUS 2-STAGED PROCEDURES

Midfoot dislocation often goes undetected in the neuropathic patient. This situation can lead to chronic foot deformity with risk of ulceration. If the injury is identified in the acute phase, the soft tissues have not shortened significantly. There is also no associated bone in callus formation and thus a closed reduction and percutaneous fixation is relatively straightforward. However, missed or chronic midfoot dislocation results in shortening of the foot owing to contracture of the soft tissues. The longer the delay to diagnosis, the more likely closed reduction becomes impossible. Owing to the plantar-based position of the cuneiform is there is ongoing risk of ulceration owing to high peak pressures.

Dislocation of the metatarsals dorsally also means that the patient can find getting footwear extremely difficult owing to the depth of the midfoot. Surgical reconstruction is beneficial both to the patient's quality of life and to decrease the risk of subsequent ulceration.

Open surgery carries an increased risk regarding the soft tissue envelope. Even when significant resection of bone is performed to facilitate reduction, swelling can still be an issue. This swelling can cause significant postoperative tension on the wounds, the inability to close the soft tissue envelop, and potential wound dehiscence. There are 2 surgical options for management with minimally invasive surgery.

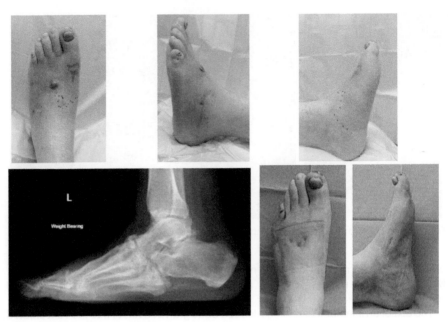

Fig. 13. Complications: Infection.

In a 2-staged reduction,[43] an external circular frame is applied and gradual reduction of the dislocation with distraction allows the soft tissues to lengthen over a period of time. The second stage procedure is performed once the soft tissues are out to length and the tarsometatarsal joints can be relocated without tension on the soft tissues. The tarsometatarsal joints are then prepared using a minimally invasive burr. Secondary fixation with intramedullary beams and bolts holds the reduction and allows the patient to be transferred to a total contact cast. The patient then has a plantigrade foot that is back to length.[43]

The challenge for the patient, however, that is that this process takes several months in the frame followed by a number of months in total contact casting. Complications such as infection were also reported at the tibial pin site, which responded to antibiotics.

Alternatively, a 1-stage minimally invasive procedure can be performed. This procedure required resection of the distal one-third of the cuneiforms/cuboid and proximal thirds of the metatarsal to allow reduction of the metatarsals. This is then held with percutaneous and beams and bolts.[29] The advantage of the single stage procedure is a single operation. However, the compromise is a shorter foot. For most patients this is not a major consideration as the foot has been bulky and deformed for a long period for time.

SUMMARY

NEMISIS has a definite role in the management of diabetic foot pathology. As minimally invasive surgical techniques for foot and ankle surgery gain wider acceptance, coupled with advances from industry in implants, customized jigs, and biologics continue to evolve, the indications and timing of minimally invasive surgery will continue to become more apparent.

As services resume after the pandemic, there is an opportunity to revisit multidisciplinary pathways to improve the escalation process for these life-changing and often life-preserving procedures. It has been a necessary consequence of the redistribution of resources of the last 2 years that complex reconstructions such as these have been delayed or put on hold. This situation has obviously been detrimental to the patient, with an increased risk of ulceration and decreased quality of life. However, there has also been a major and significant impact for training opportunities for surgeons in training to develop their surgical skills. An early return to cadaveric training laboratories and visiting fellowships is crucial to ensure that the major advances in diabetic foot surgery in the last 20 years do not regress.

DISCLOSURE

The author has nothing to disclose.

REFERENCES

1. Sun H, Saeedi P, Karuranga S, et al. IDF diabetes atlas: global, regional and country-level diabetes prevalence estimates for 2021 and projections for 2045. Diabetes Res Clin Pract 2022;183:109119.
2. Miller RJ. Neuropathic minimally invasive surgeries (NEMESIS): percutaneous diabetic foot surgery and reconstruction. Foot Ankle Clin 2016;21(3):595–627. Available at: https://www.sciencedirect.com/science/article/pii/S1083751516300377.
3. Apelqvist J, Bergqvist D, Eneroth M, et al. The diabetic foot. Optimal prevention and treatment can halve the risk of amputation. Lakartidningen 1999;96(1–2): 37–41.
4. Armstrong DG, Lavery LA. Diabetic foot ulcers: prevention, diagnosis and classification. Am Fam Physician 1998;57(6):1325–8.
5. Bakker K, Dooren J. A specialized outpatient foot clinic for diabetic patients decreases the number of amputations and is cost saving. Ned Tijdschr Geneeskd 1994;138(11):565–9.
6. Bus SA, van Netten JJ, Lavery LA, et al. IWGDF guidance on the prevention of foot ulcers in at-risk patients with diabetes. Diabetes Metab Res 2016;32: 16–24. Wiley Online Library All Journals MEDLINE (Ovid) Wiley Online Library All Journals MEDLINE (Ovid).
7. Doorgakant A, Davies MB. An approach to managing midfoot Charcot deformities. Foot Ankle Clin 2020;25(2):319–35. Available at: https://www. sciencedirect.com/science/article/pii/S108375152030022X.
8. Frykberg RG, Belczyk R. Epidemiology of the Charcot foot. Clin Podiatr Med Surg 2008;25(1):17–28. Elsevier ClinicalKey Journals MEDLINE (Ovid) Elsevier ClinicalKey Journals MEDLINE (Ovid).
9. Hingorani A, LaMuraglia GM, Henke P, et al. The management of diabetic foot: a clinical practice guideline by the society for vascular surgery in collaboration with the American Podiatric Medical Association and the Society for Vascular Medicine. J Vasc Surg 2016;63(2, Supplement):3S–21S. https://doi.org/10.1016/j.jvs. 2015.10.003. Available at: https://www.sciencedirect.com/science/article/pii/ S074152141502025X.
10. Pinzur MS, Evans A. Health-related quality of life in patients with Charcot foot. Am J Orthop (Belle Mead NJ) 2003;32(10):492–6.
11. Ragnarson Tennvall G, Apelqvist J. Prevention of diabetes-related foot ulcers and amputations: a cost-utility analysis based on Markov model simulations. Diabetologia 2001;44(11):2077–87.

12. Kennon B, Leese GP, Cochrane L, et al. Reduced incidence of lower-extremity amputations in people with diabetes in Scotland: a nationwide study. Diabetes Care 2012;35(12):2588–90.

13. Dhawan V, Spratt KF, Pinzur MS, et al. Reliability of AOFAS diabetic foot questionnaire in Charcot arthropathy: Stability, internal consistency, and measurable difference. Foot Ankle Int 2005;26(9):717–31.

14. Kroin E, Chaharbakhshi EO, Schiff A, et al. Improvement in quality of life following operative correction of midtarsal Charcot foot deformity. Foot Ankle Int 2018; 39(7):808–11.

15. Hedetoft C, Rasmussen A, Fabrin J, et al. Four-fold increase in foot ulcers in type 2 diabetic subjects without an increase in major amputations by a multidisciplinary setting. Diabetes Res Clin Pract 2009;83(3):353–7.

16. Driver VR, Fabbi M, Lavery LA, et al. The costs of diabetic foot: the economic case for the limb salvage team. J Vasc Surg 2010;52(3 Suppl):17S–22S.

17. Matricali GA, Dereymaeker G, Muls E, et al. Economic aspects of diabetic foot care in a multidisciplinary setting: A review. Diabetes Metab Res Rev 2007; 23(5):339–47.

18. Kavarthapu V. Is there a need for diabetic foot orthopaedic surgery as a sub-specialty? J Clin Orthopaedics Trauma 2021;17:72–3. Available at: https://www.sciencedirect.com/science/article/pii/S0976566221001259.

19. Botezatu I, Laptoiu D. Minimally invasive surgery of diabetic foot - review of current techniques. J Med Life 2016;9(3):249–54. JMedLife-09-249 [pii].

20. Wukich DK, Sadoskas D, Vaudreuil NJ, et al. Comparison of diabetic Charcot patients with and without foot wounds. Foot Ankle Int 2017;38(2):140–8.

21. Armstrong DG, Stacpoole-shea S, Nguyen H, et al. Lengthening of the Achilles tendon in diabetic patients who are at high risk for ulceration of the foot. J Bone Joint Surg Am 1999;81(4):535–8. Journals@Ovid Ovid Autoload MEDLINE (Ovid) Journals@Ovid Ovid Autoload MEDLINE (Ovid).

22. Greenhagen RM, Johnson AR, Bevilacqua NJ. Gastrocnemius recession or tendo-Achilles lengthening for equinus deformity in the diabetic foot? Clin Podiatr Med Surg 2012;29(3):413–24. Elsevier ClinicalKey Journals MEDLINE (Ovid) Elsevier ClinicalKey Journals MEDLINE (Ovid).

23. Brodsky JW. The diabetic foot. In: Coughlin MJ, Mann RA, Saltzman CL, editors. Surgery of the Foot and Ankle. Mosby: St. Louis; 2007. p. 1281–368.

24. Eichenholtz SN. Charcot joints. J.Bone Joint Surg 1962;44:1485.

25. Tiruveedhula M, Graham A, Thapar A, et al. Outcomes of tendo-Achilles lengthening and weight-bearing total contact cast for management of early midfoot Charcot neuroarthropathy. J Clin Orthopaedics Trauma 2021;17.

26. Sammarco GJ, Conti SF. Surgical treatment of neuroarthropathic foot deformity. Foot Ankle Int 1998;19(2):102–9.

27. Myerson MS, Kadakia AR. 10 - surgery for the neuropathic foot and ankle. In: Myerson MS, Kadakia AR, editors. Reconstructive foot and ankle surgery: management of complications. third edition. Philadelphia: Elsevier; 2019. p. 121–40. Available at: https://www.sciencedirect.com/science/article/pii/B978032349693300010X.

28. Dos Santos-Vaquinhas A, Parra G, Martínez P, et al. Beaming in the Charcot foot: a case series with 12-month minimum follow-up. Foot (Edinb) 2021;47:101814. Available at: https://www.sciencedirect.com/science/article/pii/S0958259221000407.

29. Miller R. NEMISIS minimally invasive surgical correction for midfoot Charcot arthropathy. Foot Ankle Orthopaedics 2018;3(3). 2473011418S00353.

30. Scott RT, DeCarbo WT, Hyer CF. Osteotomies for the management of Charcot neuroarthropathy of the foot and ankle. Clin Podiatr Med Surg 2015;32(3): 405–18. Elsevier ClinicalKey Journals MEDLINE (Ovid) Elsevier ClinicalKey Journals MEDLINE (Ovid).

31. Grant WP. The Journal of Foot and Ankle Surgery 2011;50(2):182–9.

32. Sammarco VJ. Superconstructs in the treatment of Charcot foot deformity: Plantar plating, locked plating, and axial screw fixation. Foot Ankle Clin 2009;14(3): 393–407.

33. Lamm BM, Siddiqui NA, Nair Ajitha K, LaPorta G. Intramedullary foot fixation for midfoot Charcot neuroarthropathy. J Foot Ankle Surg 2012;51(4):531–6. Elsevier ClinicalKey Journals MEDLINE (Ovid) Elsevier ClinicalKey Journals MEDLINE (Ovid).

34. Wiewiorski M, Yasui T, Miska M, et al. Solid bolt fixation of the medial column in Charcot midfoot arthropathy. J Foot Ankle Surg 2013;52(1):88–94. Available at: https://www.sciencedirect.com/science/article/pii/S1067251612002086.

35. Ha J, Hester T, Foley R, et al. Charcot foot reconstruction outcomes: a systematic review. J Clin Orthopaedics Trauma 2020;11(3):357–68. Available at: https://www.sciencedirect.com/science/article/pii/S0976566220301089.

36. Chraim M, Krenn S, Alrabai HM, et al. Mid-term follow-up of patients with hindfoot arthrodesis with retrograde compression intramedullary nail in Charcot neuroarthropathy of the hindfoot. Bone Joint J 2018;100-B(2):190–6. Journals@Ovid Ovid Autoload Journals@Ovid Ovid Autoload.

37. Baker JR, Glover JP, McEneaney PA. Percutaneous fixation of forefoot, midfoot, hindfoot, and ankle fracture dislocations. Clin Podiatr Med Surg 2008;25(4): 691–719. Elsevier ClinicalKey Journals MEDLINE (Ovid) Elsevier ClinicalKey Journals MEDLINE (Ovid).

38. Biz C, Ruggieri P. Minimally invasive surgery: osteotomies for diabetic foot disease. Foot Ankle Clin 2020;25(3):441–60.

39. Butt DA, Hester T, Bilal A, et al. The medial column synthes midfoot fusion bolt is associated with unacceptable rates of failure in corrective fusion for Charcot deformity. Bone Joint J 2015;97-B(6):809–13.

40. Brandão RA, Weber JS, Larson D, et al. New fixation methods for the treatment of the diabetic foot: beaming, external fixation, and beyond. Clin Podiatr Med Surg 2018;35(1):63–76.

41. Richter M, Mittlmeier T, Rammelt S, et al. Intramedullary fixation in severe Charcot osteo-neuroarthropathy with foot deformity results in adequate correction without loss of correction - results from a multi-centre study. Foot Ankle Surg 2015;21(4): 269–76.

42. Lyons M, McGregor PC, Pinzur MS, et al. Risk reduction and perioperative complications in patients with diabetes and multiple medical comorbidities undergoing Charcot foot reconstruction. Foot Ankle Int 2021;42(7):902–9.

43. Klag EA, Fisk FE, Maier LM, et al. Staged percutaneous treatment of a complete Lisfranc dislocation secondary to Charcot arthropathy: a case report. JBJS Case Connect 2021;11(4).

Etiology, Epidemiology, and Outcomes of Managing Charcot Arthropathy

Thomas Hester, MBBS, MSc, FRCS(Tr&Orth),
Venu Kavarthapu, FRCS(Tr&Orth)*

KEYWORDS

• Charcot • Neuroarthropathy • Etiology • Epidemiology • Reconstruction
• Outcomes

KEY POINTS

• In the presence of peripheral neuropathy, a swollen, red, and warm foot can be due to Charcot neuroarthropathy.
• Intense inflammatory reaction triggered by the Charcot process can lead to fragmentation of bones, instability of joints, and damage to the ligaments, resulting in foot deformity.
• The key outcome of treatment of Charcot foot is to achieve a shoeable, plantigrade and stable foot that allows weight-bearing with no risk of ulceration.

INTRODUCTION

Jean-Martin Charcot (**Fig. 1**) first described the entity in patients with tertiary syphilis in 1868, and Sir James Paget noted it as a distinct pathologic entity, naming the process "Charcot disease."[1] It has subsequently been associated with diabetes, spinal cord injuries, alcoholic peripheral neuropathy, and Charcot-Marie-Tooth disease.[2,3] Charcot neuroarthropathy (CN) has a negative impact on the quality of life of patients, with approximately 50% of patients requiring at least one operation of the foot, and in the presence of ulceration and infection an amputation rate is seen of between 35% and 67%.[4–6] The aim of this article is to provide an overview of the cause, epidemiology, and the outcomes including the associated costs of management.

ETIOLOGY

There is no single cause for the development of CN and is likely to be multifactorial. However, there are 2 well-accepted hypotheses of the pathogenesis, neurotraumatic

Kings College Hospital, Denmark Hill, London SE5 9RS, United Kingdom
* Corresponding author. Consultant Orthopaedic Surgeon, Kings College Hospital, Denmark Hill, London SE5 9RS, United Kingdom
E-mail address: venu.kavarthapu@nhs.net

Foot Ankle Clin N Am 27 (2022) 583–594
https://doi.org/10.1016/j.fcl.2022.03.002
1083-7515/22/Crown Copyright © 2022 Published by Elsevier Inc. All rights reserved.

foot.theclinics.com

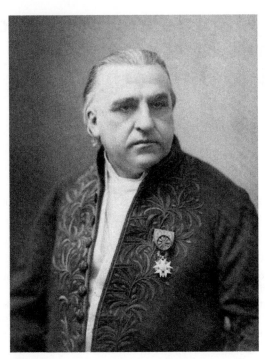

Fig. 1. Jean-Martin Charcot.

and neurovascular theories.[7–9] The neurotraumatic theory is based on repetitive microtrauma in a limb that has loss of protective sensation (LOPS). When LOPS is present, the initial traumatic incident activates the Charcot process. The response to the trauma is with an acute-phase release of proinflammatory cytokines, tumor necrosis factor alpha (TNFα), interleukin-1β, and interleukin-6. TNFα upregulates the receptor activator of nuclear factor-κB ligand (RANKL) system, which is responsible for an increase in osteoclastogenesis resulting in excessive bone turnover, whereas there is a decrease in antiinflammatory cytokines, interleukin-4 and interleukin-10, and osteoprotegerin, which is the antagonist to RANKL.[10–12] The activation of the RANKL pathway causes substantial bone resorption and fragility, increasing the risk of pathologic fracture. The heightened inflammatory reaction and hyperglycemic environment in diabetes denatures and weakens tendons and ligaments (nonenzymatic glycosylation), further destabilizing the mechanical environment.[13] The end result is fragility and instability of the bones, joints, and ligaments in a foot that has LOPS, which leads to collapse and deformity.

The neurovascular theory, first described by Charcot, proposes a state of hyperemia generated from alterations in the sympathetic nervous system, which increases venous pressure. The increased pressure compromises tendons and ligaments in the foot and ankle leading to joint instability.[14] In addition, the hyperemia may directly cause increased bone resorption by the increased delivery of osteoclasts and monocytes, resulting in greater osteoclastic activity in this area.[9] These hypotheses also go some way to explain the finding that patients with a Charcot foot show increased blood flow to the area, whereas patients with peripheral arterial disease and diabetes are relatively protected from developing Charcot; however, they still shed little light on why Charcot knee or shoulder can occur in isolation.[15,16]

Continued weight-bearing in the presence of LOPS and without the use of protective strategies (ie, total contact casting or reduced weight-bearing) perpetuates the course of repetitive microtrauma. This further increases the delivery of proinflammatory cytokines, magnifies the intensity of the Charcot process, and prevents normal bone remodeling in the affected area. This repetitive process to the bones and joints exceeds the structural integrity, leading to fracture, subluxation, or dislocation and associated deformity. The competing process of destruction and repair favors bone resorption.[17] More recent molecular studies continue to support an early inflammatory process in CN but do not show a uniform decline in described markers even after treatment.[18] The role of calcitonin gene–related peptide (CGRP) that is normally secreted from nerve terminals in the regulation of the inflammatory response has recently been investigated. CGRP is known to antagonize the synthesis of RANKL; hence a reduction of CGRP due to nerve damage can lead to an increase in RANKL expression. Faster fracture resolution was noted in a small cohort of Charcot foot patients managed with a single dose of RANKL antibody.[19] A better understanding of the interplay between these complex pathways and common genetic polymorphisms among those affected by CN is required to fully understand its pathogenesis.[20–23]

EPIDEMIOLOGY

The incidence of Charcot has been reported as between 0.3% and 0.85% annually among people with type 2 diabetes. The actual incidence may vary by ethnicity or geographic location, with different incidences reported for non-Hispanics and Mexican Americans, although this may be partly due to a failure to recognize the diagnosis.[24–26] It was recognized that some regional differences identified globally were due to lack of consistency in the choice of disease codes used for CN. One study from Italy showed that different international disease codes, based on the original clinic presentations, were used to record newly diagnosed CN.[27]

The prevalence of CN is largely unknown, as extensive population studies are not available; however, estimates range from 0.08% of the general diabetes patient population to 13% of patients presenting at a high-risk diabetic foot clinic.[24,25] It occurs most commonly in the fifth decade of life and in greater than 80% of those who have suffered from diabetes for more than 10 years. The demographics are different among patients with type 1 and type 2 diabetes. The peak age of CN affection is lower among those with type 1 (peak at third and fourth decade) in comparison to type 2 (peak at sixth and seventh decade).[28] The duration of diabetes before developing CN is longer among patients with type 1 diabetes compared with type 2. The condition is bilateral in 10% of patients.[13,29,30]

OUTCOMES OF MANAGEMENT

The technical aspects of nonoperative and operative management of Charcot are complex and falls outside the remit for this article. What all treatments have in common is to achieve the following outcomes: limb salvage, structural stability of the foot and ankle, infection eradication, ulceration prevention, and restoration of a plantigrade foot. These can be achieved with operative and nonoperative methods.

Broadly speaking, a major amputation in patients with diabetes is not a risk-free procedure with predictable outcomes. The 1- to 2-year mortality following transtibial amputation in the overall diabetic population is between 25% and 36%.[31–33] The overall data may be skewed with the suggestion that diabetic patients who undergo amputation for gangrene are more likely to die than those who undergo amputation for infection or failure following attempted reconstruction. One must also remember that the average body mass index of the patients undergoing limb reconstruction for Charcot foot is greater than 35.[33]

OUTCOMES AFTER SURGICAL RECONSTRUCTION

No standardized outcome measure has been identified for neuropathic feet.[34] However, the American Orthopaedic Foot and Ankle Society scores being most widely used, demonstrate overall improvement with fixation of approximately 38 points (**Figs. 2** and **3**).[35–40] Time to weight-bearing was reached in a mean of 17 weeks.[37,40–57]

Fusion Rates

Charcot-affected bones show less healing response, and the bone fusion rates following reconstructions are typically low. More recent studies have utilized

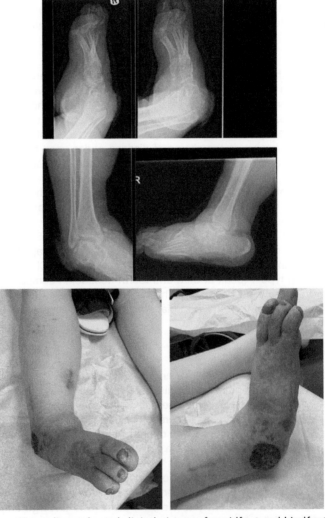

Fig. 2. Preoperative radiographs and clinical picture of a midfoot and hindfoot deformity.

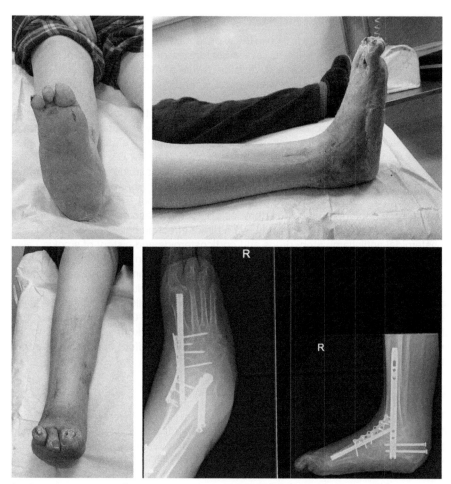

Fig. 3. Postoperative radiographs and clinical pictures of a complex reconstruction.

advanced fixation techniques in the surgical reconstruction of Charcot deformities that may improve the fusion outcomes. Fusion rates are seen as an important surgical outcome measure; the overall fusion rate in Charcot reconstructions in one systematic review has been shown to be 86%.[34] However, there was significant heterogeneity within the methodology of recording fusion rates from clinical to radiological union. Moreover, CN fusion rates reported in recent studies included more complex reconstructions with complex deformities, impaired distal limb circulation, and osteomyelitis (OM). Earlier series from Papa and colleagues[58] in 1993 showed only a 30% union rate of tibiocalcaneal (posttalectomy) fusions compared with a 90% tibiotalar union rate. Garapati and colleagues,[59] in 2004, reported 90.5% fusion rate in 21 feet, with ulcerations in 8, whereas Dalla Paola, in 2007, reported 77.8% fusion rate in a series of 18 patients with hindfoot CN without ulceration, managed with hindfoot nail.[60] Vasukutty, in 2018, reported a 97% fusion rate among 42 hindfoot corrections with preoperative ulcerations noted in 23 feet.[61] The likely reason for the variability in reporting of fusion rates is because a nonunion is not necessarily a cause to intervene, as multiple studies found the fibrous nonunions to be stable sufficient to achieve a positive functional result and not require any addition surgery.[62]

Complication Rates and Risk Factors

The overall complication rate is high in these patients, with rates quoted between 25% and 70%, with a recent systematic review demonstrating an overall rate of 36%.[34,63] Complications included amputation, revision, failure of metal work, superficial, deep and pin site infection, removal of metal work, wound dehiscence, and a reulceration rate of 6.5%.[34]

Elmarsafi and colleagues[64] looked at a large retrospective case series to identify specific risk factors associated with major lower extremity amputation after diabetic Charcot reconstruction. The risk factors with the highest statistical significance were postreconstructive nonunion, the development of a new CN site, and the presence of PAD. Other important risk factors were renal disease, delayed postoperative healing, development of postoperative OM, and elevated HbA1c. Nonunion rates in patients with diabetes mellitus are higher than those without. There are many factors that influence fracture healing and arthrodesis outcomes. Diabetes mellitus, peripheral arterial disease, and hypothyroidism have a direct effect on bone healing. The use of nonsteroidal antiinflammatory drugs and corticosteroids and history of smoking also have a direct deleterious effect on bone healing.[65] Nonunion rates also require more robust fixation, increased diligence toward anatomic alignment, and an increased postoperative period of immobilization.[66] Metal work failures are also distinctly more common among CN reconstructions. Kummen and colleagues[67] have identified 19 hardware failures among 78 patients who had undergone CN reconstructions. This study revealed that a body mass index of greater than 30 kg/m^2 contributed to 3.5 times the risk of hardware failure, whereas combined hindfoot and midfoot reconstructions to 12 times.

Postsurgical Reconstruction Amputation Rate

The reported postreconstruction amputation rates are low, with overall amputation rates at 5.0%. The only large study assessing risk factors for a major amputation following reconstruction identified peripheral arterial disease, renal disease, delayed postoperative healing, postoperative wound infection, postoperative OM, transfer ulceration, new site of Charcot collapse, and postreconstruction nonunion for a postreconstruction amputation.[34] Surgical trauma can induce a new onset of acute CN. When this occurs, hardware from the previous surgical reconstruction can become infected because of new ulcer recurrence. Increased derangement of the foot and ankle essentially translates into increased infection of the soft tissue and bone, leading to a strong association with major amputation. Elmarsafi and colleagues looked to further quantify which factors had an increased likelihood of amputation. Renal disease has also been shown to confer a 3.7-fold increased likelihood for major amputation. A delay in soft tissue healing of greater than 30 days after the index closure is associated with a 2.6 times increased likelihood of major amputation. The development of postoperative OM imparts a 2.4-fold increased likelihood for major amputation.[64]

Published limb salvage rates are variable, and this generally reflects the variation in the complexity of presentations and the multidisciplinary support provided to the patients. One study, published in 2012, on 45 feet had a limb salvage rate of 78% following reconstruction.[68] Pinzur and Kelikia reported a series of 178 patients with a limb salvage rate of 95.7%.[46] Siebachmeyer and colleagues,[69] in 2015, reported a 100% limb salvage among 21 Charcot hindfoot reconstructions performed using internal fixation technique, whereas Vasukutty, in 2018, from the same unit, also reported 100% limb salvage among 42 hind foot corrections with preoperative ulcerations in 23 feet.[61]

COST COMPARISON

From a health system perspective, patients with severe Charcot foot deformity, with or without bony infection, pose a notable drain on available health care resources. It is known that the cost of diabetic foot ulcers places a great economic burden on society, both to health care costs and loss of productivity.[70] It is also evident that the number of people with diabetes is expected to increase over the coming decades, likely bringing with it an increasing number of associated Charcot and deformity-related foot issues. The cost of operative correction of deformity on the long-term therapeutic footwear must be weighed against the encumbered activity restriction of accommodative bracing. With the extensive complication rates including multiple surgeries, prolonged rehabilitation, and still the possibility of reulceration or amputation, inevitably health economics become an important question. Comparative effectiveness financial models are beginning to be used to assist health care systems in decision-making on allocation of resources. The economic cost of management of diabetic foot ulcers is huge. The cost in 2014 to 2015 is estimated at between £837 million and £962 million in the United Kingdom, which accounted for 0.8% of the National Health Service Budget for England and an astonishing $71 billion cost in the United States for 2017.[70,71]

   With the aim of eradication of diabetic foot ulcers, there is an increasing trend for surgical correction and limb salvage rather than amputation. There is a widely held belief that successful correction of the acquired deformity allows patients more independence to greatly improve quality of life and foster greater walking independence, which leads to a longer survival, compared with both the impaired quality of life associated with encumbered bracing and that of a transtibial amputee.[31,32] The traditional or historical view suggests that the surgery is not justified, given the cost of care and risks associated with the surgery. Although the short-term 12-month health care–related costs look very similar at $56.712 for salvage versus $49,251 for amputation.[33] The long-term costs may be more significant; if mobility is decreased after amputation and the need for social care increases due to the immobility, then the real cost benefit of limb salvage may be reached. The 1- to 2-year mortality following transtibial amputation in the overall diabetic population is between 25% and 36%.[32]

   Fleischer and colleagues[72] looked at the optimal cost-effective therapeutic approach for people suffering with unstable Charcot arthropathy of 3 competing treatment strategies for adults suffering with unstable, midfoot Charcot arthropathy. When comparing the cost-effectiveness of transtibial amputation, Charcot reconstruction, and lifetime bracing, it was found that lifetime bracing was cost-effective in all clinical scenarios. Charcot reconstruction was also cost-effective in the nonulcerated and ulcerated scenarios and offered the greatest potential for maximal quality-adjusted life-years gained.

DISCUSSION

CN is a debilitating condition. The associated foot and ankle deformity has a dramatic negative affect on lifestyle, leading to frequent negative impact on health-related quality of life for affected individuals, leading to both substantial disability and resource consumption.[34] The goals of management are to obtain a stable, plantigrade, ulcer free foot, with minimal disruption to the patient; this can only be achieved with a multidisciplinary approach and appropriate techniques. These final points are essential, as aforementioned complications are inevitable when dealing with this high-risk group of patients and as such, we as health care professionals must also remain reticent to the associated health care costs with the management of CN.

CLINICS CARE POINTS

- CN has a negative impact on the quality of life of patients.
- Infected ulceration of Charcot foot carries an amputation rate of 35% to 67%.
- The 1- to 2-year mortality following transtibial amputation in the overall diabetic population is between 25% and 36%.
- The pathophysiology of CN involves activation of the RANKL pathway contributing to bone resorption and fracture.

DISCLOSURE

The authors have nothing to disclose.

REFERENCES

1. Charcot MJ. Sur quelques arthropathies qui paraissent dependre d'une lesion du cerveau ou de la moelle epiniere. Arch Physiol Norm Pathol 1868;1:161–78.
2. Bariteau JT, Tenenbaum S, Rabinovich A, et al. Charcot arthropathy of the foot and ankle in patients with idiopathic neuropathy. Foot Ankle Int 2014. https://doi.org/10.1177/1071100714543649.
3. Frykberg RG, Belczyk R. Epidemiology of the Charcot foot. Clin Podiatr Med Surg 2008;25(1):17–28, v.
4. Game FL, Catlow R, Jones GR, et al. Audit of acute Charcot's disease in the UK: the CDUK study. Diabetologia 2012;55(1):32–5.
5. Pinzur MS. Benchmark analysis of diabetic patients with neuropathic (Charcot) foot deformity. Foot Ankle Int 1999;20(9):564–7.
6. Pakarinen TK, Laine HJ, Maenpaa H, et al. Long-term outcome and quality of life in patients with Charcot foot. J Foot Ankle Surg 2009;15(4):187–91.
7. Wukich DK, Sung W. Charcot arthropathy of the foot and ankle: modern concepts and management review. J Diabetes Its Complicat 2009;23(6):409–26.
8. Strotman PK, Reif TJ, Pinzur MS. Charcot arthropathy of the foot and ankle. Foot Ankle Int 2016. https://doi.org/10.1177/1071100716674434.
9. Chisholm KA, Gilchrist JM. The charcot joint: a modern neurologic perspective. J Clin Neuromuscul Dis 2011. https://doi.org/10.1097/CND.0b013e3181c6f55b.
10. Baumhauer JF, O'Keefe RJ, Schon LC, et al. Cytokine-induced osteoclastic bone resorption in charcot arthropathy: an immunohistochemical study. Foot Ankle Int 2006. https://doi.org/10.1177/107110070602701007.
11. Jeffcoate WJ, Game F, Cavanagh PR. The role of proinflammatory cytokines in the cause of neuropathic osteoarthropathy (acute Charcot foot) in diabetes. Lancet 2005;366(9502):2058–61.
12. Ndip A, Williams A, Jude EB, et al. The RANKL/RANK/OPG signaling pathway mediates medial arterial calcification in diabetic charcot neuroarthropathy. Diabetes 2011. https://doi.org/10.2337/db10-1220.
13. Kaynak G, Birsel O, Fatih Güven M, et al. An overview of the Charcot foot pathophysiology. Diabet Foot Ankle 2013. https://doi.org/10.3402/dfa.v4i0.21117.
14. Schaper NC, Huijberts M, Pickwell K. Neurovascular control and neurogenic inflammation in diabetes. Diabetes Metab Res Rev 2008. https://doi.org/10.1002/dmrr.862.

15. Jeffcoate WJ. Abnormalities of vasomotor regulation in the pathogenesis of the acute charcot foot of diabetes mellitus. Int J Low Extrem Wounds 2005. https://doi.org/10.1177/1534734605280447.

16. Shapiro SA, Stansberry KB, Hill MA, et al. Normal blood flow response and vasomotion in the diabetic Charcot foot. J Diabetes Its Complicat 1998;12(3):147–53.

17. Johnson JT. Neuropathic fractures and joint injuries. Pathogenesis and rationale of prevention and treatment. J Bone Joint Surg Am 1967. https://doi.org/10.2106/00004623-196749010-00001.

18. Petrova NL, Dew TK, Musto RL, et al. Inflammatory and bone turnover markers in a cross-sectional and prospective study of acute Charcot osteoarthropathy. Diabet Med 2015. https://doi.org/10.1111/dme.12590.

19. Busch-Westbroek TE, Delpeut K, Balm R, et al. Effect of Single Dose of RANKL Antibody Treatment on Acute Charcot Neuro-osteoarthropathy of the Foot. Diabetes Care 2018;41(3):e21 LP–22.

20. Folestad A, Ålund M, Asteberg S, et al. IL-17 cytokines in bone healing of diabetic Charcot arthropathy patients: a prospective 2 year follow-up study. J Foot Ankle Res 2015. https://doi.org/10.1186/s13047-015-0096-3.

21. Folestad A, Ålund M, Asteberg S, et al. Offloading treatment is linked to activation of proinflammatory cytokines and start of bone repair and remodeling in Charcot arthropathy patients. J Foot Ankle Res 2015. https://doi.org/10.1186/s13047-015-0129-y.

22. Korzon-Burakowska A, Jakobkiewicz-Banecka J, Fiedosiuk A, et al. Osteoprotegerin gene polymorphism in diabetic Charcot neuroarthropathy. Diabet Med 2012;29(6):771–5.

23. Pitocco D, Ruotolo V, Caputo S, et al. Six-month treatment with alendronate in acute charcot neuroarthropathy: a randomized controlled trial. Diabetes Care 2005. https://doi.org/10.2337/diacare.28.5.1214.

24. Frykberg RG, Belczyk R. Epidemiology of the Charcot Foot. Clin Podiatr Med Surg 2008. https://doi.org/10.1016/j.cpm.2007.10.001.

25. Fabrin J, Larsen K, Holstein PE. Long-term follow-up in diabetic Charcot feet with spontaneous onset. Diabetes Care 2000;23(6):796–800.

26. Lavery LA, Armstrong DG, Wunderlich RP, et al. Diabetic foot syndrome: evaluating the prevalence and incidence of foot pathology in Mexican Americans and non-Hispanic whites from a diabetes disease management cohort. Diabetes Care 2003;26:1435–8.

27. Anichini R, Policardo L, Lombardo FL, et al. Hospitalization for Charcot neuroarthropathy in diabetes: A population study in Italy. Diabetes Res Clin Pract 2017. https://doi.org/10.1016/j.diabres.2017.03.029.

28. Petrova NL, Foster AVM, Edmonds ME. Difference in Presentation of Charcot Osteoarthropathy in Type 1 Compared with Type 2 Diabetes. Diabetes Care 2004. https://doi.org/10.2337/diacare.27.5.1235-a.

29. Papanas N, Maltezos E. Etiology, pathophysiology and classifications of the diabetic Charcot foot. Diabet Foot Ankle 2013. https://doi.org/10.3402/dfa.v4i0.20872.

30. Trieb K. The Charcot foot: Pathophysiology, diagnosis and classification. Bone Jt J 2016. https://doi.org/10.1302/0301-620X.98B9.37038.

31. Aulivola B, Hile CN, Hamdan AD, et al. Major Lower Extremity Amputation: Outcome of a Modern Series. Arch Surg 2004. https://doi.org/10.1001/archsurg.139.4.395.

32. Pinzur MS, Gottschalk F, Smith D, et al. Functional outcome of below-knee amputation in peripheral vascular insufficiency: a multicenter review. Clin Orthop Relat Res 1993. https://doi.org/10.1097/00003086-199301000-00036.

33. Gil J, Schiff AP, Pinzur MS. Cost comparison: limb salvage versus amputation in diabetic patients with charcot foot. Foot Ankle Int 2013;34(8):1097-9.

34. Ha J, Hester T, Foley R, et al. Charcot foot reconstruction outcomes: a systematic review. J Clin Orthop Trauma 2020. https://doi.org/10.1016/j.jcot.2020.03.025.

35. Stone NC, Daniels TR. Midfoot and hindfoot arthrodeses in diabetic Charcot arthropathy. Can J Surg 2000;43(6):449-55.

36. Herscovici D, Sammarco GJ, Sammarco VJ, et al. Pantalar arthrodesis for post-traumatic arthritis and diabetic neuroarthropathy of the ankle and hindfoot. Foot Ankle Int 2011;32(6):581-8.

37. Cinar M, Derincek A, Akpinar S. Tibiocalcaneal arthrodesis with posterior blade plate in diabetic neuroarthrophy. Foot Ankle Int 2010;31(6):511-6.

38. Wiewiorski M, Yasui T, Miska M, et al. Solid bolt fixation of the medial column in Charcot midfoot arthropathy. J Foot Ankle Surg 2013;52(1):88-94.

39. Hockenbury RT, Gruttadauria M, McKinney I. Use of implantable bone growth stimulation in Charcot ankle arthrodesis. Foot Ankle Int 2007;28(9):971-6.

40. Mittlmeier T, Klaue K, Haar P, et al. Should one consider primary surgical reconstruction in charcot arthropathy of the feet? Clin Orthop Relat Res 2010;468(4):1002-11.

41. Fabrin J, Larsen K, Holstein PE. Arthrodesis with external fixation in the unstable or misaligned Charcot ankle in patients with diabetes mellitus. Int J Low Extrem Wounds 2007;6(2):102-7.

42. Garchar D, DiDomenico LA, Klaue K. Reconstruction of Lisfranc joint dislocations secondary to Charcot neuroarthropathy using a plantar plate. J Foot Ankle Surg 2013;52(3):295-7.

43. Cullen BD, Weinraub GM, Van G. Early results with use of the midfoot fusion bolt in Charcot arthropathy. J Foot Ankle Surg 2013;52(2):235-8.

44. Simon SR, Tejwani SG, Wilson DL, et al. Arthrodesis as an early alternative to nonoperative management of charcot arthropathy of the diabetic foot. J Bone Jt Surg Am 2000;82-A(7):939-50.

45. El-Gafary KA, Mostafa KM, Al-Adly WY. The management of Charcot joint disease affecting the ankle and foot by arthrodesis controlled by an Ilizarov frame: early results. J Bone Jt Surg Br 2009;91(10):1322-5.

46. Pinzur MS, Kelikian A. Charcot ankle fusion with a retrograde locked intramedullary nail. Foot Ankle Int 1997;18:699-704.

47. Rooney J, Hutabarat SR, Grujic L, et al. Surgical reconstruction of the neuropathic foot. Foot 2002;12:213-23.

48. Dalla Paola L, Brocco E, Ceccacci T, et al. Limb salvage in Charcot foot and ankle osteomyelitis: combined use single stage/double stage of arthrodesis and external fixation. Foot Ankle Int 2009;30(11):1065-70.

49. Hegewald KW, Wilder ML, Chappell TM, et al. Combined internal and external fixation for diabetic charcot reconstruction: a retrospective case series. J Foot Ankle Surg 2015;55(3):619-27.

50. Caravaggi CMF, Sganzaroli AB, Galenda P, et al. Long-term follow-up of tibiocalcaneal arthrodesis in diabetic patients with early chronic charcot osteoarthropathy. J Foot Ankle Surg 2012;51:408-11.

51. Pawar A, Dikmen G, Fragomen A, et al. Antibiotic-coated nail for fusion of infected charcot ankles. Foot Ankle Int 2013;34(1):80-4.

52. Assal M, Stern R. Realignment and extended fusion with use of a medial column screw for midfoot deformities secondary to diabetic neuropathy. J Bone Jt Surg Am 2009;91(4):812–20.
53. Eschler A, Ulmar B, Mittlmeier T, et al. Combined intra- and extramedullary fixation for Charcot arthropathy – a promising concept? Injury 2015;44:S19.
54. Matsumoto T, Parekh SG. Midtarsal Reconstructive Arthrodesis Using a Multi-Axial Correction Fixator in Charcot Midfoot Arthropathy. Foot Ankle Spec 2015; 8(6):472–8.
55. Early JS, Hansen ST. Surgical reconstruction of the diabetic foot: a salvage approach for midfoot collapse. Foot Ankle Int 1996;17(6):325–30.
56. Sammarco VJ. Superconstructs in the treatment of charcot foot deformity: plantar plating, locked plating, and axial screw fixation. Foot Ankle Clin 2009;14(3): 393–407.
57. Sammarco GJ, Conti SF. Surgical treatment of neuroarthropathic foot deformity. Foot Ankle Int 1998;19(2):102–9.
58. Papa J, Myerson M, Girard P. Salvage, with arthrodesis, in intractable diabetic neuropathic arthropathy of the foot and ankle. J Bone Jt Surg Am 1993;75(7): 1056–66.
59. Garapati R, Weinfeld SB. Complex reconstruction of the diabetic foot and ankle. Am J Surg 2004;187(5A):81S–6S.
60. Dalla L, Volpe A, Varotto D, et al. Use of a retrograde nail for ankle arthrodesis in Charcot neuroarthropathy: a limb salvage procedure. Foot Ankle Int 2007;28(9): 967–70.
61. Vasukutty N, Jawalkar H, Anugraha A, et al. Correction of ankle and hind foot deformity in Charcot neuroarthropathy using a retrograde hind foot nail—The Kings' Experience. Foot Ankle Surg 2018. https://doi.org/10.1016/j.fas.2017. 04.014.
62. Farber DC, Juliano PJ, Cavanagh PR, et al. Single stage correction with external fixation of the ulcerated foot in individuals with Charcot neuroarthropathy. Foot Ankle Int 2002;23(2):130–4.
63. Dayton P, Feilmeier M, Thompson M, et al. Comparison of complications for internal and external fixation for charcot reconstruction: a systematic review. J Foot Ankle Surg 2015;54(6):1072–5.
64. Elmarsafi T, Anghel EL, Sinkin J, et al. Risk Factors Associated With Major Lower Extremity Amputation After Osseous Diabetic Charcot Reconstruction. J Foot Ankle Surg 2019. https://doi.org/10.1053/j.jfas.2018.08.059.
65. Wukich DK, Joseph A, Ryan M, et al. Outcomes of ankle fractures in patients with uncomplicated versus complicated diabetes. Foot Ankle Int 2011;32(2):120–30.
66. Bibbo C, Lin SS, Beam HA, et al. Complications of ankle fractures in diabetic patients. Orthop Clin North Am 2001;32(1):113–33.
67. Kummen I, Phyo N, Kavarthapu V. Charcot foot reconstruction—how do hardware failure and non-union affect the clinical outcomes? Ann Jt 2020. https://doi.org/ 10.21037/aoj.2020.01.06.
68. DeVries JG, Berlet GC, Hyer CF. A retrospective comparative analysis of Charcot ankle stabilization using an intramedullary rod with or without application of circular external fixator–utilization of the Retrograde Arthrodesis Intramedullary Nail database. J Foot Ankle Surg 2012;51(4):420–5.
69. Siebachmeyer M, Boddu K, Bilal A, et al. Outcome of one-stage correction of deformities of the ankle and hindfoot and fusion in Charcot neuroarthropathy using a retrograde intramedullary hindfoot arthrodesis nail. Bone Jt J 2015. https://doi. org/10.1302/0301-620x.97b1.34542.

70. Armstrong DG, Swerdlow MA, Armstrong AA, et al. Five year mortality and direct costs of care for people with diabetic foot complications are comparable to cancer. J Foot Ankle Res 2020. https://doi.org/10.1186/s13047-020-00383-2.
71. Kerr M, Barron E, Chadwick P, et al. The cost of diabetic foot ulcers and amputations to the National Health Service in England. Diabet Med 2019. https://doi.org/10.1111/dme.13973.
72. Fleischer AE, Albright RH, Armstrong DG, et al. 1151-P: A Cost-Effectiveness Analysis of Charcot Reconstruction, Transtibial Amputation, and Lifetime Bracing for Adults with Midfoot Charcot Arthropathy. Diabetes 2020;69(Supplement 1): 1151.

Nonoperative Treatment of Charcot Neuro-osteoarthropathy

Felix W.A. Waibel, MD*, Thomas Böni, MD

KEYWORDS

- Charcot arthropathy • Charcot neuro-osteoarthropathy • Charcot foot
- Nonoperative • Conservative • Treatment • Management

KEY POINTS

- Offloading and activity reduction remains the gold standard of acute Charcot neuro-osteoarthropathy treatment.
- Once inactive, Charcot neuro-osteoarthropathy should be treated with orthopedic footwear.
- The type of footwear depends on the localization and the severity of deformity.
- Current evidence does not support pharmaceutical therapy.

INTRODUCTION

Charcot neuro-osteoarthropathy (CN) has been described more than two and a half centuries ago.[1] Until today, the pathophysiology is not fully understood.[2] Presence of neuropathy is an indispensable condition.[3,4] The cause of neuropathy is diabetes in about 75%.[5] Among patients with diabetic neuropathy, the prevalence of CN is 0.09% to 1.4%.[6] The goal of CN treatment is to maintain a plantigrade, ulcer-free foot and to assure walking ability.[2,7] Therapy strategies have changed from bed rest, compressing bandages, and casts in the nineteenth century to half-and-half conservative and operative management in a tertiary referral center setting.[8,9] Most agree that active CN should be managed conservatively with reduction of physical activity and—more important—off-loading of the affected lower extremity.[2,7,8,10–14] Off-loading is usually continued until swelling, erythema, and hyperthermia have resolved.[2,14,15] It is usually necessary for up to 6 months, although there are rare reports of up to 2 years.[5,7,14,16] After resolution of CN activity, treatment should be continued with accommodative footwear to protect the mostly distorted foot from

Division of Technical and Neuroorthopaedics, Department of Orthopaedic Surgery, Balgrist University Hospital, Forchstrasse 340, Zürich 8008, Switzerland
* Corresponding author.
E-mail address: felix.waibel@balgrist.ch

Foot Ankle Clin N Am 27 (2022) 595–616
https://doi.org/10.1016/j.fcl.2022.05.002
1083-7515/22/© 2022 The Author(s). Published by Elsevier Inc.
foot.theclinics.com

ulcers and reactivation, whereas the type of footwear heavily relies on national reimbursement guidelines and patients' individual funds.[5,17]

Pathophysiology

The pathophysiology of CN is subject of chapter 5 in this issue and is therefore not further discussed in this article. However, it is important to know that often an inflammation-producing event (sprain, fracture, infection or surgical procedure) precedes CN development.[12,18]

Classifications

Three types of classifications for CN have been established in the literature. Disease activity can be classified according to the modified Eichenholtz classification (**Table 1**). Eichenholtz originally described 3 stages based on clinical findings and radiologic changes.[19] Later, those 3 stages were complemented by a prodromal stage 0 by Shibata and colleagues that demonstrates clinical findings of an active Charcot foot without radiological changes in conventional radiographs but with MRI changes.[20] Despite being criticized for several limitations (subjectivity, neglect of the anatomic distribution, neglect of patients symptoms, and comorbidities), the Eichenholtz classification is still widely used to guide treatment of CN.[21] The region affected by CN is classified by topographic classifications such as the Sanders (**Table 2**) or the Brodsky (**Table 3**) classification with the former being mostly used.[22,23] A classification aiming to serve as a prognostic tool was proposed by Rogers and colleagues.[24] The investigators created a 2-axis system containing both

Table 1			
Eichenholtz classification[19] with modifications by Shibata and colleagues[20] and Yu and Hudson[147]; adapted from Doorgakant and Davies[12]			
Stage	Description	Clinical Features	Imaging
0 (Shibata) 0 (Yu)	Prodromal stage	Inflamed foot Neuropathic foot with trauma	Radiographs: normal MRI: bone edema, stress fractures, soft tissue edema, joint effusion
1	Fragmentation (acute phase)	Warmth (>2°C c/f unaffected side), erythema, swelling Onset of deformity	Radiographs: disorganization of joints with bone debris, subchondral fragmentation, periarticular fractures, subluxations, and dislocations Osteopenia
2	Coalescence (subacute phase)	Reduced warmth (<2°C compared with (c/f) unaffected side), erythema and swelling Progression or maintenance of deformity	Radiographs: fine debris resorption, new callus formation, coalescence of fractures, periarticular sclerosis
3	Consolidation (chronic phase)	Resolution of warmth, erythema, and swelling Consolidation of deformity	Radiographs: consolidation of fractures and remodeling of bones. Reduction of sclerosis

Table 2
Sanders and Frykberg anatomic classification, adapted from Doorgakant and Davies[12]; the data from the original publication of Sanders and Frykberg[23] and the most recent report from Gratwohl et al.[5] illustrate that the anatomic distribution remains relatively stable

Type	Location	Frequency, % Sanders et al[23]	Frequency, % Gratwohl et al[5]
1	Forefoot	15	14
2	Tarsometatarsal joint	40	47
3a	Naviculocuneiform/ talonavicular/ calcaneocuboid joints	30	30
3b	Ankle/subtalar joints	10	6
4	Calcaneus	5	3

anatomic location and severity of CN (**Fig. 1**). To date, only a small case series demonstrated an increasing amount of limb loss with increased severity of CN.[25]

Diagnostic Approach and Clinical Findings

The diagnosis of CN is challenging but crucial to start with an appropriate treatment. Before referral to a foot and ankle specialist, up to 95% of cases are missed.[26] A combination of medical history, physical examination, and imaging is necessary to establish the correct diagnosis.

The medical history should cover the following questions because they help to estimate the probability of CN and to guide diagnostics:

- Effective date of the onset of clinical symptoms (swelling, erythema)
- Presence of a preceding, potentially inflammatory producing event
- Presence of diabetes mellitus and effective date of its diagnosis (usually, CN occurs 8–12 years after diagnosis of diabetes mellitus[27])
- Presence of neuropathy and prior consultations of a neurologist
- Presence of potential risk factors for CN (obesity, ages 55–64 years, diabetes duration 6 years or more, hemoglobin A_{1c} 7% or more, renal failure, arthritis, patients who have undergone pancreas-kidney transplant, and deficiency anemia[28,29])

The clinical presentation depends on CN activity. A clinically active Charcot foot (Eichenholtz stages 0 and I) demonstrates erythema, swelling, and warmth[5,7,30–32] (**Fig. 2**). The difference in temperature compared with the contralateral, unaffected

Table 3
Brodsky anatomic classification[22] adapted from Doorgakant and Davies,[12] with data from Trepman et al.[41] and Miller[148]

Type	Location	Frequency, %
1	Tarsometatarsal/naviculo-cuneiform joints	60
2	Talonavicular/calcaneocuboid/subtalar joints	10
3a	Tibiotalar joint	20
3b	Calcaneal tuberosity	<10
4	Combination of areas	<10
5	Forefoot	<10

Classifying Charcot Arthropathy
(more proximal)

Location and Stage	1. Forefoot	2. Midfoot	3. Rearfoot/Ankle
A. Acute Charcot without deformity	Low Risk of Extremity Amputation		
B. Charcot with deformity			
C. Charcot with deformity and ulceration			
D. Charcot with osteomyelitis			High Risk of Extremity Amputation

(more complicated)

Fig. 1. Two-axis system containing both anatomic location and severity of CN proposed by Rogers and Bevilacqua.[24]

foot is 3°C to 5°C with gradual cooling when treatment has been initiated. Values given in the literature are on average 0.022°C ± 0.0005°C per day, 0.35°C per month, or 2.1°C for every 100 days.[32–35] Although manual palpation is not objective enough to assess temperature in CN, infrared dermal thermometry has been reported to be

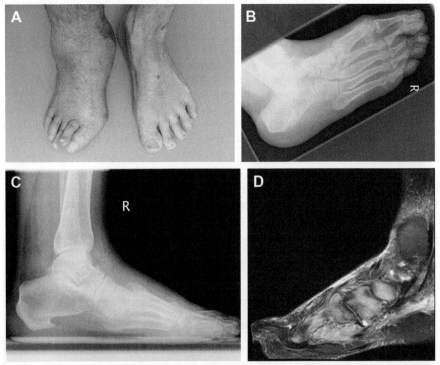

Fig. 2. Active Charcot neuro-osteoarthropathy Eichenholtz stage 1 in a 40-year-old man who is type 2 diabetic (*A*) with oblique (*B*) and lateral (*C*) radiographs. The corresponding MRI demonstrates bone edema (*D*).

reliable.[36,37] Differential diagnoses such as gout, pseudogout, erysipelas, cellulitis, deep vein thrombosis, complex regional pain syndrome (CRPS), rheumatoid arthritis, osteoarthritis, and especially osteomyelitis and septic arthritis must be considered.[30,38–40] To distinguish clinically between active CN and infection is difficult. Absence of skin lesions makes infection unlikely.[41] Furthermore, elevation of the affected extremity for several minutes leads to a decrease in erythema in case of active CN, but not in patients suffering from infection.[2,42] Systemic inflammation parameters such as C-reactive protein, white blood cell count, and erythrocyte sedimentation rate are also elevated in active CN—particularly in early stages—and therefore cannot be used to rule out infection.[43] Discrimination of the prodromal stage and Eichenholtz stage 1 is clinically difficult. Presence of deformity would indicate Eichenholtz stage 1 but can be masked by erythema and swelling. Presence of typical changes in radiographs (bony fragmentation, fractures, and joint [sub-] luxation) distinguishes between Eichenholtz stage I and the prodromal stage.[38] Transition to Eichenholtz stage II is clinically marked by a decrease in swelling and erythema and by a temperature difference of less than 2°C.[44]

Presence of neuropathy is an indispensable condition to diagnose CN.[3,4] In most cases, the 10-g Semmes-Weinstein monofilament test is sufficient to diagnose neuropathy.[45,46] In case of doubt, nerve conduction studies should be requested.[45,47] When regular nerve conduction studies are also negative and CN is clinically still strongly suspected, a neurologist should be asked for presence of small fiber neuropathy. Small fiber damage occurs early in the process of neuropathy and is associated with the presence of CN.[48] Among other tests, contact heat evoked potentials are used to test for the presence of small fiber neuropathy.[48–50]

Radiologic Findings

Radiologic workup depends on the clinical presentation. When active CN is suspected, conventional radiographs (at least a weight-bearing dorsoplantar (dp), a lateral foot, and an antero-posterior (ap) ankle radiograph) are mandatory. An MRI should be performed to confirm or exclude the prodromal Eichenholtz stage 0 when conventional radiographs are negative.[51]

Despite often being normal in the prodromal stage, conventional weight-bearing radiographs are the first step in diagnosis of CN.[30,51] As early as in Eichenholtz stage 1, typical findings as bony fragmentation, fractures and joint (sub-) luxation can be seen.[19] Furthermore, they allow assessment of angular measurements and thereby monitoring disease progression and in determining Charcot feet at risk for ulcer development.[52–54] One study reported that all patients suffering from plantar CN ulcers demonstrated a lateral-talar fist metatarsal angle of less than −27°.[53] Wukich and colleagues[55] indicated that lateral column involvement measured by a negative cuboid height contributes specifically to ulcer development, which was later questioned by results of Meyr and colleagues.[56]

MRI has several roles in the diagnosis of CN. First, it can establish an early diagnosis of Charcot foot in prodromal stages.[57] Second, it helps to monitor the course of healing and the success of off-loading and to determine switch from offloading to therapeutic footwear.[58,59] Third, it is useful in evaluation of CN complications such as osteomyelitis and soft tissue infections.[42,51] The role of CT scans is limited to surgical planning (reconstruction, removal of exostoses), whereas nuclear medicine imaging might be useful in case of suspected osteomyelitis and MRI contraindication.[51] Ultrasonography is able to detect soft tissue inflammation and bone changes before radiographic measures so that it might provide some value in the prodromal stage.[60]

Management of Charcot Neuro-osteoarthropathy

The priority of CN therapy is to maintain a stable and plantigrade foot without pain, ulcer development, and osteomyelitis.[2,17,61] The management relies on expert opinions and case series. There is a lack of randomized, controlled studies comparing conservative and surgical treatment. In the nineteenth century, CN was managed with bed rest, compressing bandages, and casts.[8] Ever since, the treatment approach has substantially changed, especially within the last 30 years. Surgical treatment has emerged in such a manner that already in 1999, 50.6% of patients referred to a tertiary care university hospital in the United States were treated surgically.[9] Among patients initially being treated conservatively, 42% needed some type of surgical therapy during follow-up in a tertiary referral center in Switzerland.[5] In the authors' opinion, nineteenth century modalities hospitalization and initial bed rest (combined with physiotherapeutic instruction) are still appropriate nowadays for a short period whenever the patient is unable to adhere with off-loading and protected weight-bearing.

Active CN (or Eichenholtz stages 0 to II) is managed conservatively by most investigators with reduction of physical activity and off-loading until resolution of activity symptoms.[5,14,15,31,58,62–67] When CN activity has resolved, patients are fitted with commercially available depth-inlay shoes and custom-made insoles/footbeds.[7,68,69] Nevertheless, continuous conservative management of CN is often impossible. Surgical treatment of CN is addressed in chapter 7 of this issue. In brief, surgical treatment is indicated[30,61,69–75] whenever there is

- A severe deformity with an open wound and osteomyelitis,
- A severe deformity with an open wound refractory to off-loading,
- A severe midfoot or hindfoot deformity with instability,
- A severe deformity with recurrent ulcers despite initial healing with off-loading.

Treatment of Active Charcot Neuro-osteoarthropathy (Prodromal Stage and Eichenholtz Stages I and II)

Initiation of treatment

Whenever active CN is suspected or diagnosed, immediate off-loading to prevent development or worsening of CN deformity should be started combined with a decrease in physical activity.[5,14,15,31,58,62–67,76,77] Early off-loading in case of the prodromal stage has been reported to prevent secondary CN deformity.[78,79] Contrarily, treatment delay leads to an increase in progressive deformities followed by complications such as ulcers, infection, and an enhanced necessity of secondary surgical procedures.[26] Those clinical findings are supported by 2 studies that demonstrated an increase of proinflammatory cytokines (inyerleukin [IL]-6 and tumor necrosis factor-α; IL-17A, IL-17E, and IL-17F) after off-loading initiation, and accelerated bone healing on radiographs.[80,81] The rationale is that off-loading activates an inflammatory stage and thereby contributes to bone remodeling.[80]

In patients unable to comply with off-loading due to insecurity with the off-loading device, even short hospitalization and instruction physiotherapy should be considered to ensure patient adherence to the offloading regime. Besides the risk of developing or worsening of CN deformity development without off-loading,[82] one study reported that failing to adhere to the off-loading regime is a significant risk factor for CN recurrence (odds ratio 19.7).[83]

Type of off-loading device

An irremovable total contact cast (TCC) is the preferred off-loading device throughout the literature[5,7,17,18,31,58,84,85] (**Fig. 3**). It is custom molded and maintains contact with

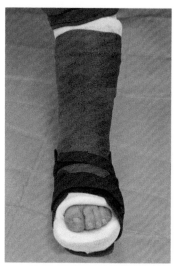

Fig. 3. Irremovable total contact cast.

the entire surface of the planta pedis and the entire lower limb therefore minimizing pressure distribution to the foot.[39,86] The TCC reduces plantar foot pressures and swelling and maintains patient mobility.[84,86,87] The downfall of TCC is that it is labor intensive and needs an experienced technician for fabrication.[86] Furthermore, because it reduces swelling rapidly, frequent outpatient visits and TCC changes are necessary (initially weekly).[14,30,58,86] Besides adaption of the TCC due to reduction in swelling, those visits also serve to detect skin lesions potentially stemming from the TCC.[14,64,88,89] Guyton described an overall complication rate of 5.52% when using the TCC in patients with diabetes or idiopathic neuropathy, mainly ulcers.[88] CN was present in slightly more than half of the cohort and associated with the highest risk (odds ratio 1.46) of developing complications.[88] Of note, the TCC can also be used as a removable device (**Fig. 4**).[58]

A second option is the instant total contact cast (iTCC). iTCC consists of a removable walker that is secured with a layer of tape or fiberglass and therefore made irremovable.[90,91] Lower costs and easier application compared with TCC have been reported.[30]

The third option are prefabricated or custom-made removable walkers such as the Charcot restraint orthotic walker (CROW) (**Fig. 5**). These walkers seem to be equally effective in off-loading but carry the downfall of lesser patient adherence.[65,87,92–94] Complications reported are pressure-related pain, ulcers, and pressure-induced muscular atrophy of the calf with subsequent malfunction.[87,95] These walkers are contraindicated in patients with a substantial amount of volume fluctuation because this can compromise fit and functionality of the off-loading device.[96] One study reported a poor outcome combining the CROW with early weight-bearing in terms of major amputation (14.9%) and ulcer development (64.9%).[62] Generally, irremovable devices seem to calm down CN activity quicker than removable devices.[97–99]

The fourth option are ankle foot orthoses (AFOs) that are built individually based on a cast positive of the affected limb. The orthosis is fabricated in a multistep procedure and consists of polyethylene terephtalate glycol (PETG) that is transparent and therefore allows for identification of remaining pressure spots (patients' skin turns red in

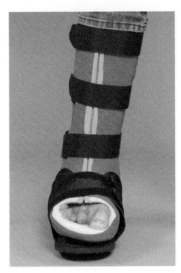

Fig. 4. Removable total contact cast.

remaining pressure spots upon donning) and their immediate elimination using a hot air gun. As the final step, the PETG is reinforced with carbon fibers. Koller and colleagues stated that the AFO was intended and used for patients with active CN but restricted their report to 200 patients who were fitted after surgical correction of CN.[95] In the authors' practice, AFOs are fabricated after initial TCC treatment when the amount of swelling is stable and are combined with compression stockings to maintain a stable volume of the affected limb. In the authors' opinion, they are particularly useful in Eichenholtz stage 2.

Weight-bearing

Persistent weight-bearing seems to cause poor outcomes in terms of limb loss and inability to walk.[82] Non-weight-bearing was historically used but seems unnecessary.[8,82] However, the literature now suggests that continued weight-bearing while

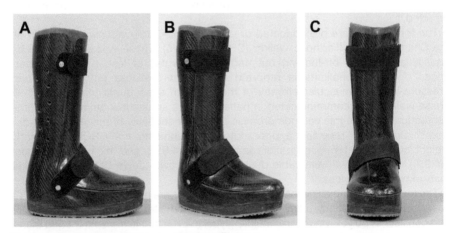

Fig. 5. (A–C) Charcot restrained orthotic walker.

using an off-loading device allows acute CN to dissolve and to maintain a stable and plantigrade foot.[14–16,39,98] Dodd and Daniels concluded that protected weight-bearing with an irremovable device seems to be the safest approach in the treatment of acute CN.[2]

Duration of off-loading

The predominant recommendation throughout the literature is to maintain off-loading until swelling and erythema have regressed and the difference in temperature is < 2° C compared with the unaffected foot.[14–16,32,67,100] Off-loading is usually necessary for up to 6 months, although there are rare reports of up to 2 years off-loading.[5,7,14,16,101] Relying on clinical signs only seems to be associated with a certain amount of CN reactivation.[32,67] The reason is possibly a longer yet subtle disease process, which is demonstrated by longer persistence of MRI changes than clinical signs of CN. Therefore, some suggest leaning on resolution of MRI changes when deciding to stop off-loading.[18,59,102,103] One study reported that the mean healing time was 6.8 ± 2.3 months for clinical signs and 8.3 ± 2.9 for resolution of MRI changes.[102] Furthermore, MRI changes seem to fluctuate over the disease course, which must be considered when MRIs are interpreted.[59] Infrared thermometry was used in 2 studies to objectify temperature reduction of less than 2.2°C compared with the unaffected limb besides reduction of erythema and swelling.[35,104] Moura-Neto and colleagues[35] reported zero reactivations within 1 year using this strategy while not reporting possible other complications. Armstrong and Lavery[104] reported that increased temperature gradients may be predictive of future ulcers. Wu and colleagues[105] proposed Doppler spectrum analysis as a tool that may reflect CN activity, but to date, there are no studies testing their hypothesis. One study described that a duration of off-loading greater than or equal to 90 days can be predicted using a score (Balgrist Score) deriving from MRI changes.[106] Being published in 2021, there are no studies that have tested the score in larger population. In summary, there is lack of evidence that clearly supports one method to evaluate the optimal timepoint to discontinue off-loading.[107]

Treatment of Inactive Charcot Neuro-osteoarthropathy (Eichenholtz Stage 3)

When CN activity has resolved, the goal is to provide the patient with footwear that prevents the foot from ulcers and bone injury (and thereby CN reactivation) by relief of pressure or peak forces.[18,64] The importance of protective footwear is underlined by plantar pressure measurements. Several studies reported of peak plantar pressure elevation in patients suffering from CN.[108,109]

Pressure Reduction with Orthopedic Footwear

Different amounts of pressure reduction have been described for the different elements that are contained in orthopedic footwear: insoles and shoe modifications. The results mainly focus on forefoot (including metatarsal head region) and heel. In the forefoot region, insoles and shoe modifications are additive (reaching pressure reduction of 30%–40%), whereas they counteract one another in the heel region.[110]

Drerup[111] investigated the effect of custom-molded multidurometer foot orthoses and shoes modified with a forefoot rocker and a midfoot rocker with and without a stiff sole. The investigators demonstrated that when compared with a flat cork insole, peak plantar pressure of the forefoot was reduced to 75.9% using the custom-molded multidurometer foot orthosis alone, to 77.4% using a midfoot rocker with a stiff sole, and to 53.6% using a combination of both. The heel demonstrated peak plantar pressure reduction to 71% using all 3 modalities. In contrast, the midfoot demonstrated peak plantar pressure elevation with the 3 modalities named before. Peak plantar pressure in the midfoot region increased less when a forefoot rocker was used instead of a midfoot rocker.[111] Zwaferink and colleagues[112] published similar results when comparing 3 types of data-driven custom-made footwear concepts, including orthopedic custom-made shoes. In contrast to both cited studies before, Keukenkamp and colleagues[109] demonstrated that plantar midfoot pressures in CN can be reduced by 80% when wearing custom-made footwear.

Position of the apex and angular orientation of rocker soles have been investigated in several studies. Chapman and colleagues[113] reported that the apex of the rocker sole should not be placed more distally than at 60% of shoe length and that the rocker angle should not go less than 20° for optimal pressure reduction. The same working group specified that placement of the apex at 52% of shoe length in combination with a rocker angle of 20° would be optimal for pressure reduction in the forefoot.[114]

Use of a carbon reinforcement for maximizing shoe outsole bending stiffness significantly reduces peak pressures underneath the metatarsal heads while increasing peak pressures underneath the heel.[115]

A shank extension is believed to further unload the plantar aspect of the patient's foot by circumferential loading of the lower limb and by limitation of foot and ankle motion.[96,116–118] However, Praet and Louwerens[119] could not demonstrate a significant plantar pressure reduction when using a shank twice the lateral malleolar height.

Choice of Orthopedic Footwear

Patients are fitted with commercially available depth-inlay shoes combined with either off-the-shelf or multidurometer foot orthoses in some countries and a stiff walking sole including a rocker bottom.[7,18,68,69] Choice of off-the-shelf or custom-made multidurometer foot orthoses depends on the presence of plantar deformities.[96]

In some countries in Europe the artisanal orthopedic shoemaker is still available because their products are covered by health insurances for CN among other indications.[5,18,75,120,121] Existence of orthopedic shoemakers allows physicians to fit patients with individualized orthopedic shoes, which are either prefabricated and then individualized (orthopedic serial shoe) or produced according to an individualized last in a multistep process that usually takes at least 2 to 6 weeks (orthopedic custom-made shoe)[18,122] (Fig. 6). Orthopedic serial shoes can be used in the absence of severe foot and ankle deformities. Orthopedic custom-made shoes are reserved for severe deformities.[122] Both modalities include a stiff walking sole, a rocker bottom, and multidurometer foot orthoses. Use of an extended shank is particularly useful in case of severe deformities and residual coronal plain instability of the ankle and/or subtalar joint. Fitting is further possible after surgical correction of CN and depends on the remaining deformity.[74,75] Availability of those individualized orthopedic shoes might contribute to a more successful conservative management of CN with less complications than in environments where this artisanal is not available. However, this is an assumption of the authors, and there are no studies comparing conservative management with commercially available depth-inlay shoes and custom accommodative foot orthoses versus individualized orthopedic shoes. When orthopedic shoemakers are unavailable, usage of complex bracing techniques such as AFOs or CROWs as a permanent solution is also possible.[17] Physicians must expect restricted patients' adherence to complex and bulky footwear.[7,122,123]

Several retrospective studies have evaluated the outcome of conservative treatment of CN and reported a high amount of complications. Ulcers occur in 37% to 72%,[5,62–64,66,67,124–126] and ulcer recurrence occurs in 40% to 49%.[5,63,64] Reactivation of CN has been reported in 7% to 33%.[5,66,67,83,127] Any CN-related surgical

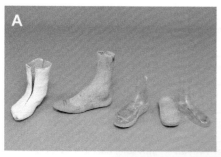
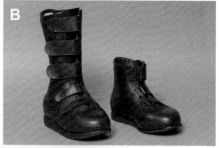
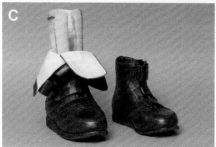

Fig. 6. Orthopedic custom-made shoe. (*A*) (*From left to right*) The cast negative of the affected foot, the last, and the foil sample shoe. The foil sample shoe allows shoemaker and physician to identify and correct remaining pressure points after production of the last. (*B*) One pair of orthopedic custom-made shoes, the right side with CN has an extended shank. (*C*) The shank extension after removal of the external leather.

procedure was performed in 42% to 56%.[5,63,64,124] Ultimately, limb loss occurred in 1% to 15%.[5,62–64,66,67,124] Those numbers illustrate the severity of CN impressively. **Table 4** summarizes the footwear usually prescribed in the authors' daily practice. This concept contributed to the results of conservative CN treatment published by Gratwohl and colleagues.[5] **Fig. 7** demonstrates the treatment algorithm of CN used by the authors, which has been adapted from Sanders and colleagues.[128]

Process of Fitting Orthopedic Footwear

Fitting of any orthopedic device in Eichenholtz stage 3 depends on volume stability of the affected limb.[18] Despite resolution of CN activity, edema in Eichenholtz stage 3 patients is often present and due to physical inactivity and/or comorbidities. Volume fluctuation can lead to nonfitting orthopedic devices and pressure ulcers. Therefore, the patient must be checked for volume fluctuation and, if present, treated by compression stockings.[18] A crucial timepoint is the transfer from the off-loading device to final footwear because the off-loading device (especially the TCC) often contributes to volume containment. Often, when the patient omits the TCC, edema quickly develops. Thus, once the transfer has been executed, special attention should be directed at volume fluctuations.

Furthermore, transfer from the off-loading device (ie, TCC) to the final orthopedic device should be seamless. Even after delivery of the final orthopedic device, the patient should be instructed to keep his TCC initially. The rationale is that (non-) customized orthopedic devices can contain pressure points that may lead to pressure ulcers.[18] In consequence, during the process of wearing in the new device, the patient should

Table 4
Choice of orthopedic footwear according to the Sanders classification in the authors practice

Sanders Type	Shoe Type	Modifications
1	Orthopedic serial or custom-made shoe[a]	Stiff sole, forefoot rocker, and custom-molded footbed
2	Ankle-high orthopedic serial or custom-made shoe[a]	Stiff sole, midfoot rocker, and custom-molded footbed
3	Ankle-high orthopedic serial or custom-made shoe[a]	Stiff sole, midfoot rocker, and custom-molded footbed
4	Orthopedic custom-made shoe[b] with an extended shaft (height: 3 times the distance of sole of foot to medial malleolus)	Stiff sole, backspaced rocker, and custom-molded footbed
5	Orthopedic custom-made shoe[b] with an extended shaft (height: 3 times the distance of sole of foot to medial malleolus)	Stiff sole, backspaced rocker, and custom-molded footbed with targeted heel offloading

The results presented by Gratwohl et al. rely on this algorithm.[5]

[a] Choice of serial or custom-made shoe is made at the discretion of both the prescribing orthopedic surgeon and the fabrication orthopedic shoemaker and depends on deformation severity.

[b] Hindfoot deformities usually make fitting of an orthopedic serial shoe impossible as the shank extension needs to be individualized.

- Wear in the new device *for 20 to 30 minutes only* during the first few days and rely on the TCC for the rest of the day,
- Perform *daily controls* of his affected limb himself after wearing the new device to rule out new pressure points,
- *Be controlled daily* by a relative or by nursing staff in case of patient retinopathy or unreliability,
- *Gradually increase* wearing in time after 3 to 4 days when there is no sign of any new pressure point (to double wearing in time is reasonable), and
- *Be controlled frequently on an outpatient basis* (depending on patients' adherence to the management during active CN, those controls should be made every 2–4 weeks initially).[18,122]

Furthermore, physician and orthopedic shoemaker/pedorthist should decide together what adaptions should be made in case of pressure points or new ulcers.[122,129]

The Role of Pharmaceutical Therapy

The role of pharmaceutical therapy in addition to off-loading is debated in the literature. According to the limited knowledge of CN pathophysiology, antiresorptive agents (bisphosphonates) were evaluated. Use of zoledronate led to an increased total time of immobilization,[130] but this finding was not confirmed in a second study.[131] Pain and temperature reduction were reported for the use of bisphosphonates.[132,133] Das and colleagues[131] reported that use of methylprednisolone significantly increased the total immobilization time. A RANKL inhibitor (denosumab) in combination with a TCC demonstrated a significantly decreased total immobilization time as opposed to TCC treatment alone.[134] Despite some promising results, a systematic review and meta-analysis from 2021 concluded that the limited evidence does not support the role of antiresorptive or anti-inflammatory drugs for earlier remission in addition to off-loading in active CN.[135]

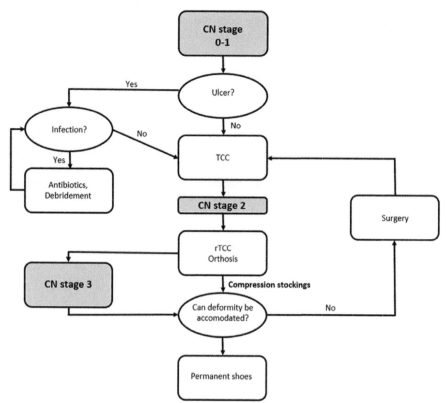

Fig. 7. Treatment algorithm of CN used by the authors, adapted from Sanders et al.[128]. rTCC, removable total contact cast.

Further Considerations

Influence of gait on plantar pressure

One possibility to further reduce plantar pressure is to adapt gait. In general, increasing velocity increases plantar pressure in the heel and in the toe region, whereas a small decrease can be seen in the midfoot region. The increase is smaller when patients use custom-molded multidurometer foot orthoses and stiff soles.[136] Drerup and colleagues[137] demonstrated a significant reduction in patients with CN using step-to-gait in the forefoot area of the leading foot and in the heel area of the contralateral foot. Also, they demonstrated that reducing stride length by 23% leads to a significant reduction of plantar pressure in all foot regions aside from the toes.[138]

Influence of bodyweight on plantar pressure

Weight reduction might contribute to plantar pressure reduction. Generally speaking, obesity leads to increased plantar pressure,[139–141] whereas weight loss reduces plantar pressure.[142] Bariatric surgery contributes to plantar pressure reduction.[143] One study found that peak plantar pressure was even a linear function of weight with weight increase leading to increased peak plantar pressures at the metatarsophalangeal joints and the heel, and vice versa.[144]

Contralateral foot

A recent study has investigated the clinical outcome of the unaffected contralateral foot in CN. The investigators reported high contralateral complication rates and suggested immediate protection of the contralateral foot with accommodative footwear.[120] Their suggestion is yet to be tested by further studies.

Peripheral arterial disease (PAD)

As opposed to prior assumptions, presence of PAD should be evaluated because it seems to come along with worse treatment outcomes.[145,146]

SUMMARY

Conservative treatment of CN is stage and deformity dependent. Acute CN is managed by off-loading and activity restriction until resolution of CN activity. There is a lack of prospective, randomized controlled studies investigating the optimal type of off-loading device, the optimal weight-bearing regime, and the best clinical-radiological definition of resolution of CN activity. Inactive CN is managed by orthopedic footwear. The type of footwear depends on the severity of CN deformity and on the presence of instability. Similar to management of active CN, there is a lack of prospective, randomized controlled studies concerning the optimal footwear once CN is inactive. A substantial amount of complications coming along with footwear treatment must be expected.

CLINICS CARE POINTS

- Start treatment immediately when Charcot arthropathy is suspected to prevent foot deformity and ulcer development.
- Use a total contact cast or a Charcot walker for off-loading while treating active Charcot arthropathy Eichenholtz stage 1.
- Use protected weight-bearing. Non-weight-bearing is not necessary, and patients with Charcot arthropathy are often unable to comply.
- Consider an AFO once the patient has transferred into Eichenholtz stage 2.
- Consider using repeat MRIs to judge resolution of Charcot activity and to guide cessation of off-loading treatment. Relying on clinical signs of activity alone may lead to increased Charcot arthropathy reactivation.
- Ensure a seamless transfer from off-loading to orthopedic footwear and pay attention to volume fluctuation of the affected limb; they can lead to malfitting of orthopedic footwear.
- Let the extent and the location of Charcot arthropathy deformity guide the choice of orthopedic footwear.
- Protect the contralateral foot immediately with orthopedic footwear because it is subject of a high number of complications.

DISCLOSURE

The authors have nothing to disclose.

REFERENCES

1. Charcot J-M. Sur quelques arthropathies qui paraissent dependre d'une lesion du cerveau ou de la moelle epiniere. Arch Physiol Norm Pathol 1868;1:161–78.
2. Dodd A, Daniels TR. Charcot Neuroarthropathy of the Foot and Ankle. J Bone Joint Surg Am 2018;100(8):696–711.

3. Koeck FX, Bobrik V, Fassold A, et al. Marked loss of sympathetic nerve fibers in chronic Charcot foot of diabetic origin compared to ankle joint osteoarthritis. J Orthop Res 2009;27(6):736–41.

4. Jeffcoate W. The causes of the Charcot syndrome. Clin Podiatr Med Surg 2008; 25(1):29–42, vi.

5. Gratwohl V, Jentzsch T, Schöni M, et al. Long-term follow-up of conservative treatment of Charcot feet. Arch Orthop Trauma Surg 2021. https://doi.org/10. 1007/s00402-021-03881-5.

6. Frykberg RG, Belczyk R. Epidemiology of the Charcot foot. Clin Podiatr Med Surg 2008;25(1):17–28, v.

7. Strotman PK, Reif TJ, Pinzur MS. Charcot Arthropathy of the Foot and Ankle. Foot Ankle Int 2016;37(11):1255–63.

8. Ramanujam CL, Zgonis T. The Diabetic Charcot Foot from 1936 to 2016: Eighty Years Later and Still Growing. Clin Podiatr Med Surg 2017;34(1):1–8.

9. Pinzur MS. Benchmark analysis of diabetic patients with neuropathic (Charcot) foot deformity. Foot Ankle Int 1999;20(9):564–7.

10. Kavitha KV, Patil VS, Sanjeevi CB, et al. New Concepts in the Management of Charcot Neuroarthropathy in Diabetes. Adv Exp Med Biol 2021;1307:391–415.

11. Schmidt BM. Clinical insights into Charcot foot. Best Pract Res Clin Rheumatol 2020;34(3):101563.

12. Doorgakant A, Davies MB. An Approach to Managing Midfoot Charcot Deformities. Foot Ankle Clin 2020;25(2):319–35.

13. Petrova NL, Edmonds ME. Conservative and Pharmacologic Treatments for the Diabetic Charcot Foot. Clin Podiatr Med Surg 2017;34(1):15–24.

14. Pinzur MS, Lio T, Posner M. Treatment of Eichenholtz stage I Charcot foot arthropathy with a weightbearing total contact cast. Foot Ankle Int 2006;27(5): 324–9.

15. Parisi MC, Godoy-Santos AL, Ortiz RT, et al. Radiographic and functional results in the treatment of early stages of Charcot neuroarthropathy with a walker boot and immediate weight bearing. Diabet Foot Ankle 2013;4. https://doi.org/10. 3402/dfa.v4i0.22487.

16. de Souza LJ. Charcot arthropathy and immobilization in a weight-bearing total contact cast. J Bone Joint Surg Am 2008;90(4):754–9.

17. Pinzur M. Surgical versus accommodative treatment for Charcot arthropathy of the midfoot. Foot Ankle Int 2004;25(8):545–9.

18. Chantelau E, Kimmerle R, Poll LW. Nonoperative Treatment of Neuro-Osteoarthropathy of the Foot: Do We Need New Criteria? Clin Podiatr Med Surg 2007;24(3):483–503.

19. Eichenholtz S. Charcot joints. Springfield (IL): Charles C. Thomas; 1966.

20. Shibata T, Tada K, Hashizume C. The results of arthrodesis of the ankle for leprotic neuroarthropathy. J Bone Joint Surg Am 1990;72(5):749–56.

21. Rosenbaum AJ, DiPreta JA. Classifications in brief: Eichenholtz classification of Charcot arthropathy. Clin Orthop Relat Res 2015;473(3):1168–71.

22. Coughlin MJ, Mann RA, Saltzman CL. Surgery of the foot and ankle. St Louis (MO): Mosby; 1999.

23. Sanders L. The Charcot foot", Levin and O'Neal's the Diabetic Foot. 5th edition. St Louis (MO): Mosby; 1993.

24. Rogers LC, Bevilacqua NJ. The diagnosis of Charcot foot. Clin Podiatr Med Surg 2008;25(1):43–51, vi.

25. Viswanathan V, Kesavan R, Kumpatla S. Evaluation of Roger's Charcot Foot Classification System in South Indian Diabetic Subjects with Charcot Foot. J Diabetic Foot Complications 2012;4:67–70.

26. Wukich DK, Sung W, Wipf SA, et al. The consequences of complacency: managing the effects of unrecognized Charcot feet. Diabet Med 2011;28(2):195–8.

27. Suder NC, Wukich DK. Prevalence of diabetic neuropathy in patients undergoing foot and ankle surgery. Foot Ankle Spec 2012;5(2):97–101.

28. Stuck RM, Sohn MW, Budiman-Mak E, et al. Charcot arthropathy risk elevation in the obese diabetic population. Am J Med 2008;121(11):1008–14.

29. Zhao HM, Diao JY, Liang XJ, et al. Pathogenesis and potential relative risk factors of diabetic neuropathic osteoarthropathy. J Orthop Surg Res 2017; 12(1):142.

30. Rogers LC, Frykberg RG, Armstrong DG, et al. The Charcot foot in diabetes. Diabetes Care 2011;34(9):2123–9.

31. van der Ven A, Chapman CB, Bowker JH. Charcot neuroarthropathy of the foot and ankle. J Am Acad Orthop Surg 2009;17(9):562–71.

32. Armstrong DG, Todd WF, Lavery LA, et al. The natural history of acute Charcot's arthropathy in a diabetic foot specialty clinic. Diabet Med 1997;14(5):357–63.

33. Petrova NL, Moniz C, Elias DA, et al. Is there a systemic inflammatory response in the acute charcot foot? Diabetes Care 2007;30(4):997–8.

34. McCrory J, Morag E, Norkitis A, et al. Healing of Charcot fractures: skin temperature and radiographic correlates. Foot 1998;8(3):158–65.

35. Moura-Neto A, Fernandes TD, Zantut-Wittmann DE, et al. Charcot foot: skin temperature as a good clinical parameter for predicting disease outcome. Diabetes Res Clin Pract 2012;96(2):e11–4.

36. Dallimore SM, Puli N, Kim D, et al. Infrared dermal thermometry is highly reliable in the assessment of patients with Charcot neuroarthropathy. J Foot Ankle Res 2020;13(1):56.

37. Murff RT, Armstrong DG, Lanctot D, et al. How effective is manual palpation in detecting subtle temperature differences? Clin Podiatr Med Surg 1998;15(1): 151–4.

38. Holmes C, Schmidt B, Munson M, et al. Charcot stage 0: A review and considerations for making the correct diagnosis early. Clin Diabetes Endocrinol 2015; 1:18.

39. Schade VL, Andersen CA. A literature-based guide to the conservative and surgical management of the acute Charcot foot and ankle. Diabet Foot Ankle 2015; 6:26627.

40. Poll LW, Weber P, Böhm HJ, et al. Sudeck's disease stage 1, or diabetic Charcot's foot stage 0? Case report and assessment of the diagnostic value of MRI. Diabetol Metab Syndr 2010;2:60.

41. Trepman E, Nihal A, Pinzur MS. Current topics review: Charcot neuroarthropathy of the foot and ankle. Foot Ankle Int 2005;26(1):46–63.

42. Heidari N, Oh I, Li Y, et al. What Is the Best Method to Differentiate Acute Charcot Foot From Acute Infection? Foot Ankle Int 2019;40(1_suppl):39s–42s.

43. Hingsammer AM, Bauer D, Renner N, et al. Correlation of Systemic Inflammatory Markers With Radiographic Stages of Charcot Osteoarthropathy. Foot Ankle Int 2016;37(9):924–8.

44. Papanas N, Maltezos E. Etiology, pathophysiology and classifications of the diabetic Charcot foot. Diabet Foot Ankle 2013;4. https://doi.org/10.3402/dfa.v4i0. 20872.

45. Boulton AJ, Gries FA, Jervell JA. Guidelines for the diagnosis and outpatient management of diabetic peripheral neuropathy. Diabet Med 1998;15(6):508–14.

46. Feng Y, Schlösser FJ, Sumpio BE. The Semmes Weinstein monofilament examination as a screening tool for diabetic peripheral neuropathy. J Vasc Surg 2009; 50(3):675–82, 82.e1.

47. Pinzur MS. Diabetic peripheral neuropathy. Foot Ankle Clin 2011;16(2):345–9.

48. Malik RA. Diabetic neuropathy: A focus on small fibres. Diabetes Metab Res Rev 2020;36(Suppl 1):e3255.

49. Rosner J, Hostettler P, Scheuren PS, et al. Normative data of contact heat evoked potentials from the lower extremities. Sci Rep 2018;8(1):11003.

50. Khan A, Petropoulos IN, Ponirakis G, et al. Corneal confocal microscopy detects severe small fiber neuropathy in diabetic patients with Charcot neuroarthropathy. J Diabetes Investig 2018;9(5):1167–72.

51. Rosskopf AB, Loupatatzis C, Pfirrmann CWA, et al. The Charcot foot: a pictorial review. Insights Imaging 2019;10(1):77.

52. Hastings MK, Johnson JE, Strube MJ, et al. Progression of foot deformity in Charcot neuropathic osteoarthropathy. J Bone Joint Surg Am 2013;95(13): 1206–13.

53. Bevan WP, Tomlinson MP. Radiographic measures as a predictor of ulcer formation in diabetic charcot midfoot. Foot Ankle Int 2008;29(6):568–73.

54. Hastings MK, Sinacore DR, Mercer-Bolton N, et al. Precision of foot alignment measures in Charcot arthropathy. Foot Ankle Int 2011;32(9):867–72.

55. Wukich DK, Raspovic KM, Hobizal KB, et al. Radiographic analysis of diabetic midfoot charcot neuroarthropathy with and without midfoot ulceration. Foot Ankle Int 2014;35(11):1108–15.

56. Meyr AJ, Sebag JA. Relationship of cuboid height to plantar ulceration and other radiographic parameters in midfoot charcot neuroarthropathy. J Foot Ankle Surg 2017;56(4):748–55.

57. Ergen FB, Sanverdi SE, Oznur A. Charcot foot in diabetes and an update on imaging. Diabet Foot Ankle 2013;4. https://doi.org/10.3402/dfa.v4i0.21884.

58. Renner N, Wirth SH, Osterhoff G, et al. Outcome after protected full weightbearing treatment in an orthopedic device in diabetic neuropathic arthropathy (Charcot arthropathy): a comparison of unilaterally and bilaterally affected patients. BMC Musculoskelet Disord 2016;17(1):504.

59. Chantelau EA, Antoniou S, Zweck B, et al. Follow up of MRI bone marrow edema in the treated diabetic Charcot foot - a review of patient charts. Diabet Foot Ankle 2018;9(1):1466611.

60. Mortada M, Ezzeldin N, Hammad M. Ultrasonographic features of acute Charcot neuroarthropathy of the foot: a pilot study. Clin Rheumatol 2020;39(12):3787–93.

61. Harkin EA, Schneider AM, Murphy M, et al. Deformity and clinical outcomes following operative correction of charcot ankle. Foot Ankle Int 2019;40(2): 145–51.

62. Nilsen FA, Molund M, Hvaal KH. High incidence of recurrent ulceration and major amputations associated with charcot foot. J Foot Ankle Surg 2018;57(2): 301–4.

63. Pakarinen TK, Laine HJ, Mäenpää H, et al. Long-term outcome and quality of life in patients with Charcot foot. Foot Ankle Surg 2009;15(4):187–91.

64. Saltzman CL, Hagy ML, Zimmerman B, et al. How effective is intensive nonoperative initial treatment of patients with diabetes and Charcot arthropathy of the feet? Clin Orthop Relat Res 2005;435:185–90.

65. Christensen TM, Gade-Rasmussen B, Pedersen LW, et al. Duration of off-loading and recurrence rate in Charcot osteo-arthropathy treated with less restrictive regimen with removable walker. J Diabetes Complications 2012; 26(5):430–4.

66. Jansen RB, Jørgensen B, Holstein PE, et al. Mortality and complications after treatment of acute diabetic Charcot foot. J Diabetes Complications 2018; 32(12):1141–7.

67. Fabrin J, Larsen K, Holstein PE. Long-term follow-up in diabetic Charcot feet with spontaneous onset. Diabetes Care 2000;23(6):796–800.

68. Kroin E, Chaharbakhshi EO, Schiff A, et al. Improvement in quality of life following operative correction of midtarsal charcot foot deformity. Foot Ankle Int 2018;39(7):808–11.

69. Jones C, McCormick JJ, Pinzur MS. Surgical management of charcot arthropathy. Instr Course Lect 2018;67:255–67.

70. Sammarco VJ, Sammarco GJ, Walker EW Jr, et al. Midtarsal arthrodesis in the treatment of Charcot midfoot arthropathy. J Bone Joint Surg Am 2009;91(1): 80–91.

71. Ford SE, Cohen BE, Davis WH, et al. Clinical outcomes and complications of midfoot charcot reconstruction with intramedullary beaming. Foot Ankle Int 2019;40(1):18–23.

72. Pinzur MS. Neutral ring fixation for high-risk nonplantigrade Charcot midfoot deformity. Foot Ankle Int 2007;28(9):961–6.

73. Pinzur MS, Schiff AP. Deformity and clinical outcomes following operative correction of charcot foot: a new classification with implications for treatment. Foot Ankle Int 2018;39(3):265–70.

74. Wirth SH, Viehöfer AF, Tondelli T, et al. Mid-term walking ability after Charcot foot reconstruction using the Ilizarov ring fixator. Arch Orthop Trauma Surg 2020; 140(12):1909–17.

75. Ettinger S, Plaass C, Claassen L, et al. Surgical management of charcot deformity for the foot and ankle-radiologic outcome after internal/external fixation. J Foot Ankle Surg 2016;55(3):522–8.

76. Baglioni P, Malik M, Okosieme OE. Acute Charcot foot. Bmj 2012;344:e1397.

77. Thompson RC Jr, Havel P, Goetz F. Presumed neurotrophic skeletal disease in diabetic kidney transplant recipients. JAMA 1983;249(10):1317–9.

78. Edmonds M, Petrova N, Edmonds A, et al, editors. What happens to the initial bone marrow oedema in the natural history of Charcot osteoarthropathy? Diabetologia. New York: SPRINGER; 2006.

79. Chantelau E, Richter A, Ghassem-Zadeh N, et al. Silent" bone stress injuries in the feet of diabetic patients with polyneuropathy: a report on 12 cases. Arch Orthop Trauma Surg 2007;127(3):171–7.

80. Folestad A, Ålund M, Asteberg S, et al. Offloading treatment is linked to activation of proinflammatory cytokines and start of bone repair and remodeling in Charcot arthropathy patients. J Foot Ankle Res 2015;8:72.

81. Folestad A, Ålund M, Asteberg S, et al. IL-17 cytokines in bone healing of diabetic Charcot arthropathy patients: a prospective 2 year follow-up study. J Foot Ankle Res 2015;8:39.

82. Clohisy DR, Thompson RC Jr. Fractures associated with neuropathic arthropathy in adults who have juvenile-onset diabetes. J Bone Joint Surg Am 1988; 70(8):1192–200.

83. Osterhoff G, Böni T, Berli M. Recurrence of acute Charcot neuropathic osteoarthropathy after conservative treatment. Foot Ankle Int 2013;34(3):359–64.

84. McGill M, Molyneaux L, Bolton T, et al. Response of Charcot's arthropathy to contact casting: assessment by quantitative techniques. Diabetologia 2000; 43(4):481–4.

85. Myerson MS, Henderson MR, Saxby T, et al. Management of midfoot diabetic neuroarthropathy. Foot Ankle Int 1994;15(5):233–41.

86. Myerson M, Papa J, Eaton K, et al. The total-contact cast for management of neuropathic plantar ulceration of the foot. J Bone Joint Surg Am 1992;74(2): 261–9.

87. Verity S, Sochocki M, Embil JM, et al. Treatment of Charcot foot and ankle with a prefabricated removable walker brace and custom insole. Foot Ankle Surg 2008;14(1):26–31.

88. Guyton GP. An analysis of iatrogenic complications from the total contact cast. Foot Ankle Int 2005;26(11):903–7.

89. Chantelau E. The perils of procrastination: effects of early vs. delayed detection and treatment of incipient Charcot fracture. Diabet Med 2005;22(12):1707–12.

90. Frykberg RG, Zgonis T, Armstrong DG, et al. Diabetic foot disorders. A clinical practice guideline (2006 revision). J Foot Ankle Surg 2006;45(5 Suppl):S1–66.

91. Crews RT, Wrobel JS. Physical management of the Charcot foot. Clin Podiatr Med Surg 2008;25(1):71–9, vii.

92. Jostel A, Jude EB. Medical treatment of Charcot neuroosteoarthropathy. Clin Podiatr Med Surg 2008;25(1):63–9, vi-vii.

93. Morgan JM, Biehl WC 3rd, Wagner FW Jr. Management of neuropathic arthropathy with the Charcot Restraint Orthotic Walker. Clin Orthop Relat Res 1993;(296):58–63.

94. Mehta JA, Brown C, Sargeant N. Charcot restraint orthotic walker. Foot Ankle Int 1998;19(9):619–23.

95. Koller A, Meissner SA, Podella M, et al. Orthotic management of Charcot feet after external fixation surgery. Clin Podiatr Med Surg 2007;24(3):583–99, xi.

96. Robinson C, Major MJ, Kuffel C, et al. Orthotic management of the neuropathic foot: an interdisciplinary care perspective. Prosthet Orthot Int 2015;39(1):73–81.

97. Game FL, Catlow R, Jones GR, et al. Audit of acute Charcot's disease in the UK: the CDUK study. Diabetologia 2012;55(1):32–5.

98. Sinacore DR. Acute Charcot arthropathy in patients with diabetes mellitus: healing times by foot location. J Diabetes Complications 1998;12(5):287–93.

99. Richard JL, Almasri M, Schuldiner S. Treatment of acute Charcot foot with bisphosphonates: a systematic review of the literature. Diabetologia 2012;55(5): 1258–64.

100. Pinzur MS, Sage R, Stuck R, et al. A treatment algorithm for neuropathic (Charcot) midfoot deformity. Foot Ankle 1993;14(4):189–97.

101. Griffiths DA, Kaminski MR. Duration of total contact casting for resolution of acute Charcot foot: a retrospective cohort study. J Foot Ankle Res 2021; 14(1):44.

102. Zampa V, Bargellini I, Rizzo L, et al. Role of dynamic MRI in the follow-up of acute Charcot foot in patients with diabetes mellitus. Skeletal Radiol 2011; 40(8):991–9.

103. Schlossbauer T, Mioc T, Sommerey S, et al. Magnetic resonance imaging in early stage charcot arthropathy: correlation of imaging findings and clinical symptoms. Eur J Med Res 2008;13(9):409–14.

104. Armstrong DG, Lavery LA. Monitoring healing of acute Charcot's arthropathy with infrared dermal thermometry. J Rehabil Res Dev 1997;34(3):317–21.

105. Wu T, Chen PY, Chen CH, et al. Doppler spectrum analysis: a potentially useful diagnostic tool for planning the treatment of patients with Charcot arthropathy of the foot? J Bone Joint Surg Br 2012;94(3):344–7.

106. Berli MC, Higashigaito K, Götschi T, et al. The "Balgrist Score" for evaluation of Charcot foot: a predictive value for duration of off-loading treatment. Skeletal Radiol 2021;50(2):311–20.

107. Gooday C, Gray K, Game F, et al. Systematic review of techniques to monitor remission of acute Charcot neuroarthropathy in people with diabetes. Diabetes Metab Res Rev 2020;e3328. https://doi.org/10.1002/dmrr.3328.

108. Armstrong DG, Lavery LA. Elevated peak plantar pressures in patients who have Charcot arthropathy. J Bone Joint Surg Am 1998;80(3):365–9.

109. Keukenkamp R, Busch-Westbroek TE, Barn R, et al. Foot ulcer recurrence, plantar pressure and footwear adherence in people with diabetes and Charcot midfoot deformity: A cohort analysis. Diabet Med 2021;38(4):e14438.

110. Brinckmann P, Frobin W, Leivseth G, et al. Orthopedic biomechanics. 2nd edition. New York: Thieme; 2016. p. 496, viii.

111. Drerup B. Der Einfluss der Fußbettung und Schuhzurichtung auf die plantare Druckverteilung. Medizinisch Orthopadische Technik 2000;120(3):84–90.

112. Zwaferink JBJ, Custers W, Paardekooper I, et al. Optimizing footwear for the diabetic foot: Data-driven custom-made footwear concepts and their effect on pressure relief to prevent diabetic foot ulceration. PLoS One 2020;15(4):e0224010.

113. Chapman JD, Preece S, Braunstein B, et al. Effect of rocker shoe design features on forefoot plantar pressures in people with and without diabetes. Clin Biomech 2013;28(6):679–85.

114. Preece SJ, Chapman JD, Braunstein B, et al. Optimisation of rocker sole footwear for prevention of first plantar ulcer: comparison of group-optimised and individually-selected footwear designs. J foot Ankle Res 2017;10(1):1–10.

115. Zwaferink JBJ, Custers W, Paardekooper I, et al. Effect of a carbon reinforcement for maximizing shoe outsole bending stiffness on plantar pressure and walking comfort in people with diabetes at high risk of foot ulceration. Gait Posture 2021;86:341–5.

116. Carlson JM, Hollerbach F, Day B. A calf corset weightbearing ankle-foot orthosis design. J Prosthetics Orthotics 1991;4(1):41–4.

117. Armstrong DG, Stacpoole-Shea S. Total contact casts and removable cast walkers. Mitigation of plantar heel pressure. J Am Podiatr Med Assoc 1999;89(1):50–3.

118. Dahmen R, Haspels R, Koomen B, et al. Therapeutic footwear for the neuropathic foot: an algorithm. Diabetes Care 2001;24(4):705–9.

119. Praet SF, Louwerens JW. The influence of shoe design on plantar pressures in neuropathic feet. Diabetes Care 2003;26(2):441–5.

120. Waibel FWA, Berli MC, Gratwohl V, et al. Midterm Fate of the Contralateral Foot in Charcot Arthropathy. Foot Ankle Int 2020;41(10):1181–9.

121. Larsen K, Holstein P, editors. Stress fractures as the cause of Charcot feet. Proceedings of the first International Symposium on the diabetic foot. Amsterdam: Excerpta Medica; 1991.

122. Illgner U, Wühr J, Rümmler M, et al. [Orthopedic made-to-measure shoes for diabetics. Long-term 5-year outcome]. Orthopade 2009;38(12):1209–14.

123. Reiber GE, Smith DG, Wallace CM, et al. Footwear used by individuals with diabetes and a history of foot ulcer. J Rehabil Res Dev 2002;39(5):615–22.

124. Bariteau JT, Tenenbaum S, Rabinovich A, et al. Charcot arthropathy of the foot and ankle in patients with idiopathic neuropathy. Foot Ankle Int 2014;35(10): 996–1001.

125. Larsen K, Fabrin J, Holstein PE. Incidence and management of ulcers in diabetic Charcot feet. J Wound Care 2001;10(8):323–8.

126. O'Loughlin A, Kellegher E, McCusker C, et al. Diabetic charcot neuroarthropathy: prevalence, demographics and outcome in a regional referral centre. Ir J Med Sci 2017;186(1):151–6.

127. Rudrappa S, Game F, Jeffcoate W. Recurrence of the acute Charcot foot in diabetes. Diabet Med 2012;29(6):819–21.

128. Sanders L. The Charcot foot", Levin and O'Neal's the Diabetic Foot. 7th edition. St Louis (MO): Mosby; 2007.

129. Zamosky I. Shoe modifications in lower-extremity orthotics. Bull Prosthet Res 1964;10(2):54–95.

130. Pakarinen TK, Laine HJ, Mäenpää H, et al. The effect of zoledronic acid on the clinical resolution of Charcot neuroarthropathy: a pilot randomized controlled trial. Diabetes Care 2011;34(7):1514–6.

131. Das L, Bhansali A, Prakash M, et al. Effect of methylprednisolone or zoledronic acid on resolution of active charcot neuroarthropathy in diabetes: a randomized, double-blind, placebo-controlled study. Diabetes Care 2019;42(12):e185–6.

132. Jude EB, Selby PL, Burgess J, et al. Bisphosphonates in the treatment of Charcot neuroarthropathy: a double-blind randomised controlled trial. Diabetologia 2001;44(11):2032–7.

133. Pitocco D, Ruotolo V, Caputo S, et al. Six-month treatment with alendronate in acute Charcot neuroarthropathy: a randomized controlled trial. Diabetes Care 2005;28(5):1214–5.

134. Busch-Westbroek TE, Delpeut K, Balm R, et al. Effect of Single Dose of RANKL Antibody Treatment on Acute Charcot Neuro-osteoarthropathy of the Foot. Diabetes Care 2018;41(3):e21–2.

135. Rastogi A, Bhansali A, Jude EB. Efficacy of medical treatment for Charcot neuroarthropathy: a systematic review and meta-analysis of randomized controlled trials. Acta Diabetol 2021;58(6):687–96.

136. Drerup B, Hafkemeyer U, Möller M, et al. [Effect of walking speed on pressure distribution of orthopedic shoe technology]. Orthopade 2001;30(3):169–75.

137. Drerup B, Szczepaniak A, Wetz HH. Plantar pressure reduction in step-to gait: a biomechanical investigation and clinical feasibility study. Clin Biomech (Bristol, Avon) 2008;23(8):1073–9.

138. Drerup B, Kolling C, Koller A, et al. [Reduction of plantar peak pressure by limiting stride length in diabetic patients]. Orthopade 2004;33(9):1013–9.

139. Hills AP, Hennig EM, McDonald M, et al. Plantar pressure differences between obese and non-obese adults: a biomechanical analysis. Int J Obes 2001; 25(11):1674–9.

140. Birtane M, Tuna H. The evaluation of plantar pressure distribution in obese and non-obese adults. Clin Biomech 2004;19(10):1055–9.

141. Butterworth PA, Urquhart DM, Landorf KB, et al. Foot posture, range of motion and plantar pressure characteristics in obese and non-obese individuals. Gait Posture 2015;41(2):465–9.

142. Song J, Kane R, Tango DN, et al. Effects of weight loss on foot structure and function in obese adults: a pilot randomized controlled trial. Gait Posture 2015;41(1):86–92.

143. Walsh TP, Gill TK, Evans AM, et al. Changes in foot pain, structure and function following bariatric surgery. J Foot Ankle Res 2018;11(1):35.

144. Drerup B, Beckmann C, Wetz HH. [Effect of body weight on plantar peak pressure in diabetic patients]. Orthopade 2003;32(3):199–206.

145. Wukich DK, Hobizal KB, Sambenedetto TL, et al. Outcomes of Osteomyelitis in Patients Hospitalized With Diabetic Foot Infections. Foot Ankle Int 2016;37(12): 1285–91.

146. Waibel FW, Schöni M, Kronberger L, et al. Treatment failures in diabetic foot osteomyelitis associated with concomitant charcot arthropathy - the role of underlying arteriopathy. Int J Infect Dis 2022;114:15–20.

147. Yu GV, Hudson JR. Evaluation and treatment of stage 0 Charcot's neuroarthropathy of the foot and ankle. J Am Podiatr Med Assoc 2002;92(4):210–20.

148. Miller RJ. Neuropathic Minimally Invasive Surgeries (NEMESIS):: Percutaneous Diabetic Foot Surgery and Reconstruction. Foot Ankle Clin 2016;21(3):595–627.

Managing Acute Fore- and Midfoot Fractures in Patients with Diabetes

Choon Chiet Hong, MBBS, FRCSEd[a], Stefan Rammelt, MD, PhD[b],*

KEYWORDS

- Tarsometatarsal • Mid-tarsal • Instability • Deformity • Ulceration • Reconstruction
- Minimally invasive

KEY POINTS

- Few is written and investigated about the management of acute and subacute fractures and dislocations at the fore- and midfoot in patients with diabetes who are at higher risk of complications than patients with nondiabetes.
- In compliant patients with good diabetic control as evident by the HbA1c and blood glucose level trends, operative indications can be similar to patients without diabetes.
- In patients with poorly controlled diabetes with acute fractures, extreme caution with medical optimization should be exercised because these individuals are often faced with potential risks of deformity, ulceration, and amputation whether treated operatively or not. Stable internal fixation in case of surgical treatment and prolonged offloading independent of the choice of treatment is the mainstay of management in these patients.
- The main goals of treatment of manifest Charcot neuroarthropathy (CN) are to achieve a plantigrade, stable foot that is infection- and ulcer-free and ambulant with orthopedic shoes. If operative treatment is chosen for gross instability or deformity leading to ulceration or inability to walk, the concept of superconstructs in combination with prolonged protection in a well-padded total contact cast (TCC) is applied.

BACKGROUND

Diabetes mellitus is one of the most prevalent causes of death and disability affecting just under half a billion people worldwide in 2019.[1] The prevalence of diabetes globally was estimated to be 9.3% (463 million) in 2019 which will continue to rise to 10.2% (578 million) by 2030% and 10.9% (700 million) by 2045.[2] The absolute global economic burden from diabetes was projected to increase to $2.1 trillion by 2030 posing a large burden to health systems and economies[3] because patients with diabetes are known to have longer hospital stays, extensive use of health care resources and higher readmission rates due to complications.[4–9]

[a] Department of Orthopaedic Surgery, National University Hospital, 5 Lower Kent Ridge Road, Singapore 119074; [b] University Center for Orthopaedics, Trauma and Plastic Surgery, University Hospital Carl Gustav Carus at TU Dresden, Fetscherstrasse 74, Dresden 01307, Germany
* Corresponding author.
E-mail address: stefan.rammelt@uniklinikum-dresden.de

Foot Ankle Clin N Am 27 (2022) 617–637
https://doi.org/10.1016/j.fcl.2022.02.001
1083-7515/22/© 2022 Elsevier Inc. All rights reserved.

Abbreviations	
CN	Charcot neuroarthropathy
TCC	Total contact cast
T1DM	Type 1 diabetes mellitus
PVD	Peripheral vascular disease
HbA1c	Glycated hemoglobin (marker for long-term gylcemic control)
CROW	Charcot Restraint Orthotic Walker
IQR	Interquartile range
OR	Odds ratio
NIS	Nationwide inpatient sample in the United States
MIPO	Minimally-invasive plate osteosynthesis

As this number of patients with diabetes continues to grow, orthopedic surgeons will undoubtedly see more patients with diabetes in their practice as multiple studies have shown increased risks of fractures with diabetes.[7–10] In a recent publication reviewing 979 ankle fractures for more than 13 years, 13.4% of the patients had diabetes.[7] Another recent study using data from a German National Database reported a 2-fold increased all-fracture rate in patients with Type-1 diabetes mellitus (T1DM) when compared with healthy controls.[10] The cumulative all-fracture incidence was 18.4% for those with T1DM and 9.9% for patients with nondiabetes. In particular for individual fracture sites, there were statistically significant differences noted in the cumulative fracture incidence for those with fractures in the foot and toe, except ankle (ICD 10: S92%; 2.9% vs 0.7%) and lower leg including ankle (ICD 10: S82%; 3.1% vs 1.7%).[10] The cumulative fracture incidence of the foot and toe was 4-fold higher than healthy controls.[10] On top of that, a larger study in the United States with 148,483 patients from the Nationwide Inpatient Sample (NIS) database of patients with ankle fractures from 2001 to 2010 had 16.6% of their patients diagnosed with diabetes.[8] This percentage had significantly increased from an earlier study by Ganesh and colleagues using similar data from the NIS database of patients with ankle fractures from 1988 to 2000 yielding only 5.71% patients with diabetes in 160,598 patients.[9]

Patients with diabetes with foot and ankle fractures have poorer outcomes and higher risks of complications when compared with patients without diabetes.[11–15] Complications such as poor wound healing, wound infection, delayed union, malunion, nonunion, and fixation failure are commonly reported.[11–15] These arise from physiologic and metabolic abnormalities such as diabetic neuropathy, altered tissue healing, and impaired immune response.[15–18] In addition, vasculopathy in the form of peripheral vascular disease (PVD) is also a common concomitant occurrence as the incidence of PVD was reported to be 30 times more common in patients with diabetes when compared with the overall population.[19,20]

Furthermore, Charcot neuroarthropathy (CN) characterized by chronic and progressive bone and joint destruction which can lead to deformities, ulcerations, and ultimately amputations is also contributed by diabetic neuropathy.[11,12,17,18,21–23] The prevalence of CN reported ranged from 0.08% to 13% among patients with diabetes [24] and amputation risks increase significantly in patients with diabetes with CN (7 times greater risk) than those without.[23] Therefore, these distinctive features of foot and ankle fractures in patients with diabetes coupled with their physiologic and metabolic anomalies must be identified early and addressed well to reduce the risk of complications.

There is a lack of literature on the management of acute fore- and midfoot fractures in patients with diabetes, and to the best of our knowledge, there are no clinical studies on that topic. For the present review, we, therefore, have to draw similarities in treatment strategies for the ankle and hindfoot fractures in diabetics[7,11–21] coupled with own experiences to provide a systematic approach to manage these injuries. In the following, appropriate clinical assessment and 3 potential presentations with special considerations in managing the fractures of the fore- and midfoot for patients with diabetes will be discussed.

DIABETIC PHYSIOLOGIC AND METABOLIC ASSESSMENT

Appropriate clinical and medical assessment should be routinely performed for patients with diabetes with foot fractures as the management is often complex and requires a multidisciplinary approach.[11,15,20] One of the most important parameters for the evaluation of diabetes glycemic control is the glycosylated hemoglobin (HbA1c). Preoperative HbA1c should be routinely checked as studies have shown that poor glycemic control leads to high risks of wound infection and complications.[11,16,20,21,25] Wukich and colleagues have reported that an HbA1c of $\geq$ 8% leads to 2.7 times greater risks of surgical site infection when compared with those with Hba1c < 8%.[25] Ideally, the HbA1c should be well less than 8% for any elective foot and ankle surgery as it should for any acute trauma surgery. Besides, Shibuya and colleagues reported the risks of poor bone healing such as delayed union, nonunion, and malunion was strongly associated with HbA1c > 7%.[26] Perioperative blood glucose levels should also be maintained between 7.8 mmol/L and 11.1 mmol/L to reduce risks of wound infection.[11,27,28]

In patients with poorly controlled diabetes as shown by elevated HbA1c and blood glucose levels, commonly associated comorbidities such as cardiovascular disease, nephropathy, neuropathy, and compliance must be assessed and addressed before treatment with a multidisciplinary team such as a general medical internist or specialized services such as cardiology, endocrinology, nephrology and podiatrist should be initiated.[11,20] Neuropathy assessment should be performed clinically using the 5.07 Semmes-Weinstein monofilament testing which is vital to understand if the patient's protective sensation is intact as the loss of this sensation is associated with the development of neuropathic ulcerations and CN.[20,29] Vascular perfusion status should also be routinely evaluated before elective or acute trauma foot surgery. PVD itself has been shown to be an independent risk factor for periprosthetic joint infection after total ankle replacement as well as after arthrodesis procedures of the foot and ankle.[30–32] If the foot pulses are not palpable, one should consider a Doppler ultrasound which is easily available and can be conducted at the bedside to evaluate the waveforms.[20] If there are any doubts about the perfusion status, a referral to the vascular surgeons for angiography and revascularization procedure may be necessary to ensure adequate perfusion for soft tissue and bone healing. Perioperative optimization of medical comorbidities is imperative to reduce the already significantly higher risks of complications.

ACUTE FORE- AND MIDFOOT FRACTURES IN PATIENTS WITH WELL-CONTROLLED DIABETES

In compliant patients with good diabetic control as evident by the HbA1c and blood glucose level trends, operative indications can be similar to a patient without diabetes. Stable and undisplaced fractures can be treated nonoperatively although a regular shorter interval review with radiographic monitoring would be prudent. If operatively indicated, standard open reduction and internal fixation may be carried out (**Fig. 1**) favoring a minimally invasive approach if feasible to reduce any risks of wound complications (**Fig. 2**).[33] Good perioperative control of serum glucose levels is mandatory in

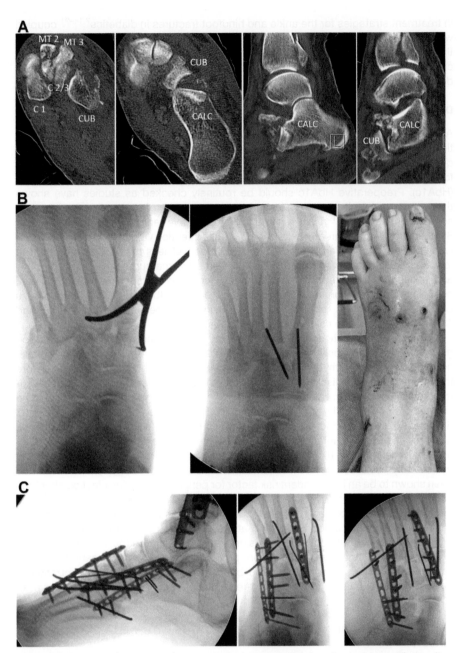

Fig. 1. (*A*) Computed tomography scans of a 68-year-old female patient with insulin-dependent diabetes mellitus showing fracture-dislocations at the ankle, mid-tarsal, and tar-sometatarsal joints after sustaining a motor vehicle accident. (*B*) With well-controlled serum glucose levels and a normal HbA1C, a staged reconstruction with internal fixation of the ankle and percutaneous gross reduction of the tarsometatarsal joint was carried out. (*C*) In-ternal fixation of the mid-tarsal and tarsometatarsal joints with bridging plates and addi-tional K-wire fixation was performed after the soft tissue swelling subsided. (*D*) At

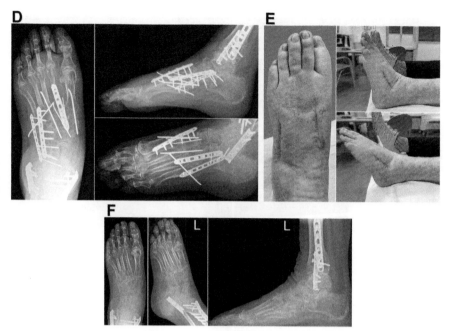

Fig. 1. (*continued*).

these patients. A recent case-control study revealed that hyperglycemia on admission, in both diabetics and nondiabetics, is an independent risk factor for deep surgical site infection and significantly associated with inferior outcomes in trauma patients.[34] Prolonged periods of casting and non-weight bearing are generally not indicated.

ACUTE FORE- AND MIDFOOT FRACTURES IN PATIENTS WITH POORLY CONTROLLED DIABETES

In patients with poorly controlled diabeteswith acute foot fractures, extreme caution with medical optimization should be stressed as the treatment of these individuals are often fraught with complications such as potential risks of deformity, ulceration, and amputation whether it is treated operatively or not.[15,20,35,36] Patients and physicians alike must be aware of the risk of new-onset CN that is triggered through an acute fracture.[12,36] Poor control of serum glucose levels may also point to poor patient compliance with respect to medication. Therefore, a thorough patient assessment including a good clinical examination of the affected foot is important. A swollen and bruised skin with blisters around the fracture should indicate high risks of soft tissue complications because patients with diabetes often display dry and fissured skin due to autonomic neuropathy.[20,37] This can give rise to cellulitis or deep infections due to the break in the epidermal layer of the skin.[20] Therefore, early reduction of a grossly displaced foot fracture and immobilization with a heavily padded cast is essential. This

---

12 weeks, the fractures are solidly healed and alignment is fully preserved. (*E*) Clinical images and sagittal range of motion at 16 weeks, 4 weeks after implant removal. (*F*) Weight-bearing radiographs at 16 weeks demonstrate anatomic midfoot and forefoot alignment with still visible disuse osteopenia from offloading.

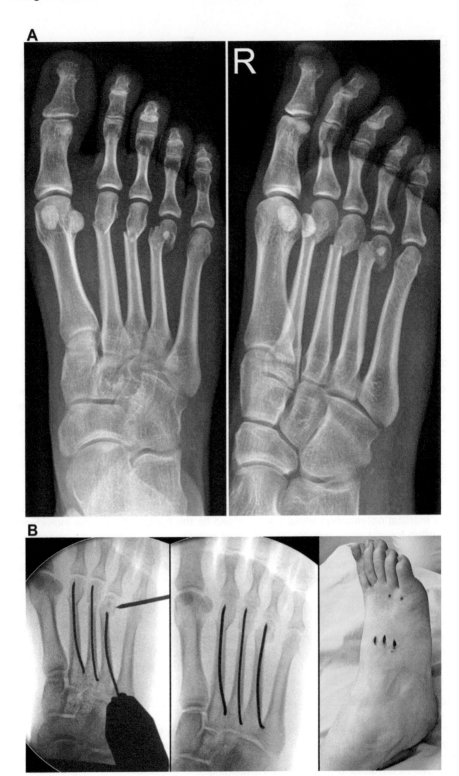

should be followed with early elevation and cooling to reduce the swelling and prevent worsening of the tissue oedema.[37] A good sign to take note would be the "wrinkle sign" as defined by the presences of wrinkles over the skin around the fracture due to the resorption of edematous fluid.[37] This can take from 7 to 14 days depending on the adequacy of immobilization and compliance to elevation.[37–39] While we are not aware of any clinical studies on the management of midfoot or forefoot fractures in diabetics, similar studies on soft tissue injuries in tibial pilon fractures have reported a delay of at least 7 to 14 days to allow for soft tissue swelling to diminish.[38,39] Sirkin and colleagues[38] who proposed staged protocol with initial external fixation followed by delayed surgical fixation of tibial pilon fracture reported an average of 12.7 days (range: 4–30 days) delay while Duckworth and colleagues[39] demonstrated a median of 7 days (IQR: 5–11 days) in their cohort of type C tibial pilon fractures treated with staged protocol.

Once the soft tissue condition is acceptable, nonoperative management can be instituted for stable and undisplaced foot fractures with a full cast for immobilization. A stable fracture boot or ankle-foot orthosis may be considered for compliant patients. Special boots with additional padding are available for patients with diabetes with neuropathy like the CROW (Charcot Restraint Orthotic Walker). A total contact cast (TCC) may be required in some cases with severe neuropathy to prevent fracture displacement and ulceration from noncompliance. The boot or cast must be taken off regularly in patients with neuropathy to check for pressure sores and avoid ulceration. The patient should also be counseled for a prolonged period of immobilization and non-weight bearing ambulation with walking aid for approximately 8 to 12 weeks. If patients are noncompliant or unable to walk on crutches to offload the affected foot due to their overall condition, immobilization in a wheelchair is preferred.

Unstable and displaced fractures should undergo early manipulation and reduction to prevent skin tenting leading to pressure ulceration. If the reduction can be held stable with a heavily padded cast, it can be treated nonoperatively with casting and regular shorter interval review. Similarly, these patients will require a prolonged period of immobilization and non-weight bearing for 8 to 12 weeks provided that there is minimal to no loss of reduction during the regular controls. However, as reported in studies on ankle fractures in patients with diabetes, one should be aware that poor outcomes are not limited to operatively treated fractures only as there is a high risk of complications following nonoperative management. Flynn and colleagues reported a 70% rate of malunion and a 66% infection rate in ankle fractures treated with closed reduction and casting.[35] Lovy and colleagues reported a 75% incidence of complications including malunion, loss of reduction, cast ulcerations, infections, and new-onset Charcot joint in their cohort of patients with diabetes with displaced ankle fractures treated nonoperatively with closed reduction and casting.[36] They concluded that nonoperative treatment was associated with a 21-fold increase in odds of complication when compared with operative treatment (75% vs 12.5%, OR 21.0, $P = .004$).[36]

Grossly unstable fractures that are refractory to closed reduction and casting but not amenable to open reduction due to critical soft tissue conditions can be held reduced with percutaneous transarticular pinning or with external fixation. For the

Fig. 2. (*A*) Serial metatarsal neck fractures with plantar deviation of the 2nd to 4th metatarsal heads in a patient with non–insulin-dependent diabetes. (*B*) Minimally invasive reduction and fixation with antegrade intramedullary wires are performed via stab incisions to prevent pathologic pressure under the metatarsal heads—that would be particularly worrisome in a diabetic patient—while minimizing possible complications from surgery.

latter, a well-tensioned fine wire (Ilizarov) fixator is preferred to minimize pin track infections. Mini-open incisions for reduction followed by percutaneous transarticular screw fixation for Lisfranc or Chopart joint fracture-dislocations can also be performed to improve construct rigidity. Following that, supplemental casting and a prolonged period of immobilization with non-weight bearing should be implemented. This group of patients can be treated definitively in this manner in an acute setting. If symptomatic arthritis develops, arthrodesis can be carried out in an elective manner once the patient is medically optimized to reduce the risks of complications.

In patients whereby the fracture pattern or presence of impending ulceration necessitates surgery, the approach should take into account both soft tissue and bony considerations. First and foremost, surgical fixation via a less extensile approach would be most appropriate to reduce soft tissue dissection and periosteal blood supply disruption with the intention to promote better soft tissue and bony healing. Mini-open incision or percutaneous screw fixations should be the routine (**Fig. 3**). Secondly, principles of internal fixation in poorly controlled diabetics should include fixation beyond fracture site into adjacent stable joints to provide stable anchors.[38] Additionally, the strongest device available for fixation should be used and applied in a mechanically advantageous fashion such as plantar plating.[40,41] It is an adaptation from the concept of "superconstructs" in stabilizing unstable foot following osteotomies in CN as described by Sammarco (**Table 1**).[40] Combination of devices such as intramedullary bolts for midfoot fractures augmented with medial or lateral column locking plates to increase construct rigidity can also be used to prevent hardware failure. Fixed angle devices such as locking plates do not rely on friction between the plate and bone providing a more rigid and stable construct when compared with non-locking plates, especially when used in osteoporotic bones which is common in patients with diabetes. Supplementation of internal fixation with minimally invasive plate osteosynthesis (MIPO) technique using locking plates to bridge the fracture site or multiple transarticular K-wire pinning and external fixation will also improve the rigidity of the fixation (**Fig. 4**). This supplementation fixation has been illustrated in multiple reports on fixation for diabetic ankle fractures whereby a more rigid construct such as multiple fibula-pro-tibia screws to increase stability of the lateral fibula fixation, large transarticular Steinmann pins through the tibiotalocalcaneal joints to maintain joint reduction while ankle malleoli heals, and external fixation augmentation have all shown improved outcomes in treating diabetic ankle fractures.[11,15–17,20,21] In our experience, such augmented fixation techniques may also be applied in a similar fashion to the fore- and midfoot fractures.

Subsequently, postoperative management such as perioperative glucose level monitoring and prolonged immobilization should be reinforced. These patients must be placed on the prolonged period of immobilization and non-weight bearing ambulation with walking aid or wheelchair for approximately 8 to 12 weeks followed by removal of external fixators or K wires and progression to protected weight bearing in a walking cast or total contact casting for another 6 weeks (**Fig. 5**). Physical therapy aims at regaining motion and minimizing edema (**Fig. 6**). As with nonoperative treatment, they should all be reviewed at regular intervals to prevent soft tissue complications such as cast ulcerations and loss of reduction.

Lastly, it is vital to recognize that a simple foot fracture can trigger the cascade of the Charcot process which can cause bone and joint destruction, bone loss, and deformity. It has been reported that trivial injury can lead to the release of proinflammatory cytokines that upregulate osteoclasts to absorb bone.[11,16–18,42–44] This bone resorption in an already neuropathic and osteopenic patient may be the stimulus for the development of CN although the development of CN is often multifactorial with other

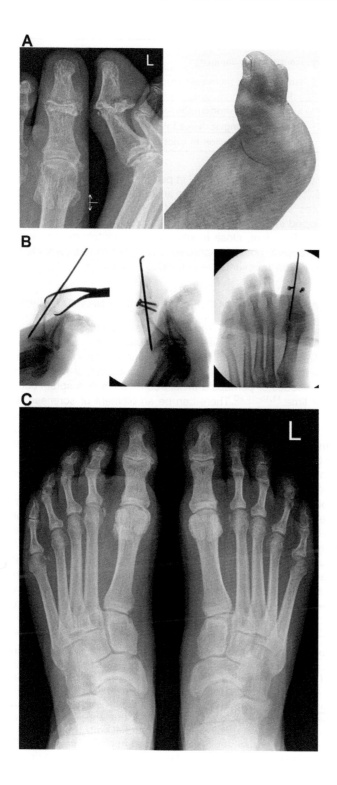

Table 1	
Criteria for "superconstruct" by Sammarco[40]	
1	Fusion beyond the osteotomy to include unaffected joints strengthens the fixation
2	Bone resection shortens the foot and reduces soft tissue tension
3	Use of the strongest device tolerated by the soft tissues
4	Application of devices in a position that maximizes mechanical function

trigger factors as the prevalence of CN in patients with peripheral neuropathy is only 0.09% to 1.4%.[18,45] Holmes and Hill when analyzing the course of 18 diabetic patients with 20 fractures and/or dislocations of the foot and ankle, found that Charcot changes developed in 8 of the 11 fractures in which there was a delay in diagnosis and treatment.[46] Therefore, close monitoring is absolutely necessary regardless of the nature of treatment (both nonoperative and operative) as early identification of a Charcot process allows preventative actions to be taken.

ACUTE FORE- AND MIDFOOT FRACTURES IN CHARCOT NEUROARTHROPATHY

It is difficult to identify acute fore- and midfoot fractures in CN as they can present to the clinician in various stages. However, one should maintain a high index of suspicion in identifying clinical features of an acute Charcot process particularly in a diabetic patient who presents with a swollen, erythematous, and hot foot with no known preceding traumatic episodes or perhaps a trivial trauma such as a sprain occurring over a short period of time.[11,15–18,20] There can be an element of soreness or pain within the foot.[11,15–18,20] In addition, it is usually unilateral with no predisposing wounds and may have been initially misdiagnosed as gout, cellulitis or thrombophlebitis.[11,17] Frequently, the patients present late after sustaining a minor trauma with increasing pain, deformity and difficulty on ambulation.

Clinical examination includes temperature measurement and a temperature difference of 2°C or more than the contralateral unaffected foot should raise suspicion of an acute process. Foot pulses should be palpated and they are characteristically bouncing due to the hyperdynamic circulation from autonomic neuropathy although some studies have shown concomitant PVD in patients with CN. Biochemical investigations usually reveal normal to mildly elevated inflammatory markers such as the white blood cell count, C-reactive protein, or erythrocyte sedimentation rate in the presence of an acute neuropathic ("Charcot") process. This is important to distinguish between an inflammatory stage of the CN versus an infectious process. In the same vein, Brodsky had also described a clinical test to differentiate a Charcot process from infection

◀━━

Fig. 3. (*A*) Grossly displaced fracture-dislocation of the right great toe in an 82-year-old male patient with diabetic polyneuropathy. Not the pressure from the displaced fragments on the base of the distal phalanx and traumatic hammertoe deformity. (*B*) Minimally invasive reduction and percutaneous screw fixation supplemented by K-wire transfixation of the IP joint was carried out together with Z-plasty of the extensor halluces longus tendon. (*C*) The patient was mobilized in a forefoot-offloading shoe and implants were removed at 10 weeks. Weight-bearing was gradually increased to full body weight until the 12th postoperative week. The toe healed stable, pain-free, and free of infection. Weight-bearing radiographs at 2 years show a stable and plantigrade great toe with some signs of arthritis at the IP joint. The patient has a limited range of motion but no pain.

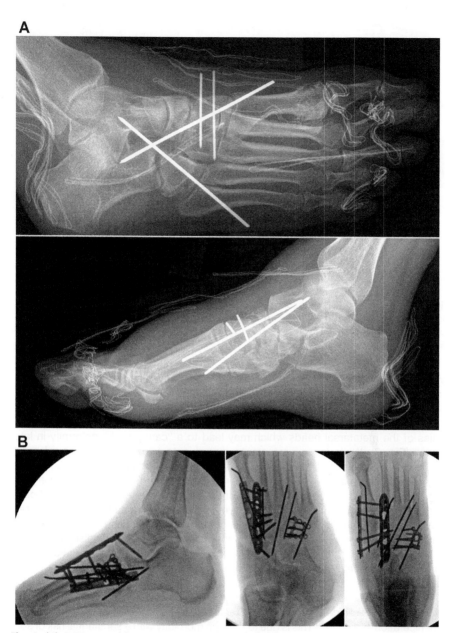

Fig. 4. (*A*) A 54-year-old woman patient with a BMI of 31 and poorly controlled, insulin-dependent diabetes is transferred from another hospital following closed reduction and K-wire transfixation of a grossly unstable fracture-dislocation at the mid-tarsal joint with navicular and cuboid fractures. (*B*) After soft tissue consolidation, internal fixation was achieved with bridge-plating of the 1st to 2nd tarsometatarsal, naviculocuneiform, and talonavicular joints and plate fixation of the fractured cuboid supplemented by K-wire transfixation.

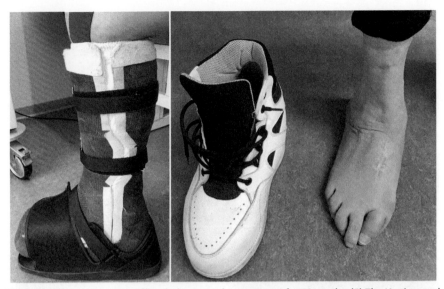

Fig. 5. (*A*) The patient was offloaded in a total contact cast for 12 weeks. (*B*) The K-wires and broken part of the dorsal bridge plate crossing the talonavicular joint were removed followed by gradual increase in weight-bearing for another 4 weeks in a customized boot. (Same patient as in **Fig. 4**).

whereby the affected lower limb is elevated for 5 to 10 minutes and if the swelling and erythema diminishes, the diagnosis of a Charcot process is supported while if the swelling and erythema persisted, it would be more likely of an infectious process.[47]

On radiographs, neuropathic fractures at the forefoot typically present with deformities of the metatarsal heads which may lead to a "candy-stick" deformity in late stages (**Fig. 7**). While these are easy to discriminate from acute metatarsal head and neck fractures in healthy bone (see **Fig. 2**), fracture-dislocations at the midfoot may mimic those in otherwise healthy patients, particularly in the tarsometatarsal joint (**Fig. 8**). However, the absence of a relevant trauma and the medical history should lead to the correct diagnosis. When analyzing 55 consecutive patients with diabetes presenting with Charcot arthropathy of the foot or ankle, Herbst and colleagues found that fracture patterns predominated at the ankle and forefoot whereas dislocations did so in the midfoot.[48] The fracture pattern was associated with peripheral deficiency of bone mineral density (BMD) whereas the dislocation pattern wasn't.[48]

In the first stage of CN whereby acute fractures and dislocations of the fore- and/or midfoot can occur, it is conventional that treatment is generally nonoperative unless there is the presence of clinical urgency such as tented skin with impending ulceration or pressure ulceration.[17,18,20,21,40] This is due to the high morbidity with a substantial risk of soft tissue and bony complications present during the acute inflammatory stage that can finally lead to major amputations. On top of that, the usual surgical challenge with treatment at the acute Stage 1 of CN is always the unclear extent of destruction and whether it will continue to progress despite fixation as it may affect adjacent joints that were considered stable initially. In addition, the bone quality during the pathogenic process of resorption and fragmentation will mostly be inadequate for fixation stability.[17,18,21,40,49] Despite some studies suggesting that early surgical intervention at Stage 1 may make fixation easier due to the more straightforward reduction and stabilization thus expediting consolidation and limiting progression to deformities,[21,50,51] most authors would concur that

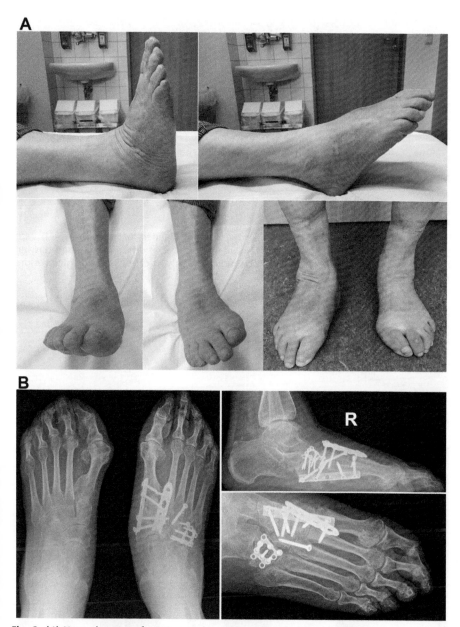

Fig. 6. (*A*) Normal range of motion at the ankle and mid-tarsal joints at 6 months. (*B*) The patient is fully weight-bearing with a stable, plantigrade foot free of ulceration despite some subsidence of the medial arch.

reconstruction, once the acute inflammatory process had ceased, have proven to be more reliable.[17,18,21,49] The need for the surgical fixation of fractures in CN seems to be higher in the ankle and hindfoot than in the fore- and midfoot.[52]

The main goals of treatment are to achieve a plantigrade, stable foot that is infection- and ulcer-free, and ambulant with orthopedic shoes. At acute Stage 1, a TCC

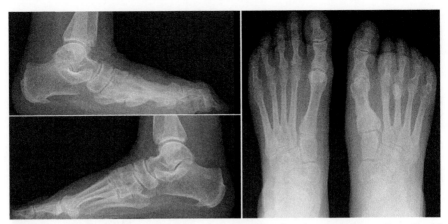

Fig. 7. Charcot neuroarthropathy (CN) at the forefoot (Sanders & Frykberg Type I) with typical deformity of all metatarsal heads including fractures of different ages and clawing of the toes. Operative treatment would be indicated only in case of pathologic pressure from grossly displaced metatarsal heads.

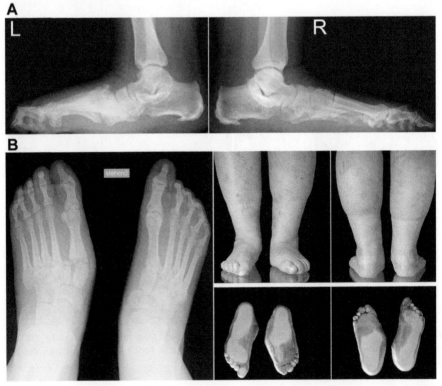

Fig. 8. (*A*) Weight-bearing radiographs of a 58-year-old obese female patient with diabetic neuropathy and increasing deformity (CN Sanders & Frykberg Type II, Brodsky Type 1), and no history of trauma, showing bilateral collapse of the foot arch. (*B*) The dorsoplantar view shows a pattern similar to a homolateral Lisfranc fracture-dislocation in the left foot. In the absence of instability or pressure ulceration, nonoperative treatment was initiated. Regular, professional foot care is warranted to prevent complications in the long term.

(see **Fig. 5**) is recommended as it helps to immobilize the joints and equalize weight distribution across the foot to prevent peak pressures at any particular point. Non-weight bearing and elevation should also be instituted for a prolonged period of up to 12 to 16 weeks with regular short interval reviews (approximate 2–3 weekly) for cast change and adjustment. Regular clinical and radiographic monitoring are also necessary to ensure prominent bony areas are well padded and fracture-dislocations are not displacing further. The patient should also be counseled and educated about the diagnosis and management plan to ensure compliance in the non-weight bearing and elevation at home.

Once the acute Charcot process in Stage 1 has progressed to Stage 2 whereby the temperature difference between the affected and contralateral foot is < 2°C and interval radiographs showed stable architecture with some callus formation, the patient can be allowed partial weight bearing with a custom molded walking cast shoe or a CROW boot with walking aids. Although the duration of immobilization and non-weight bearing can differ between individuals depending on the morphology of the foot fracture, diabetic control, and compliance, one should only initiate any form of weight bearing ambulation once the foot is considered progressively stable or already stable in Stage 3 via clinical and radiographic parameters as mentioned. Elective surgery in the form of exostectomy, osteotomy, and fusion can be undertaken later if deformity is grossly unstable or persistence of focal pressure points with ulcerations or inability to walk with orthopedic shoes.[17,18,21,40,49]

In the case of fore- and/or midfoot fractures or dislocations requiring surgery in the acute stage due to clinical urgencies such as tented skin from displaced bony fragment or pressure ulceration, mini-open reduction, and percutaneous fixation can be performed initially to reduce the risks of soft tissue complication. Following that, TCC can be resumed as per nonoperative treatment of Stage 1 CN. Alternatively, a staged surgery for internal fixation can be attempted once the patient is optimized preoperatively and the skin is not acutely swollen. Minimally invasive arthrodesis of the midfoot using intramedullary bolts can be considered after mini-open reduction and realignment of the foot columns is conducted.[53] Alternatively, open reconstruction using (additional) locking plates acting as a dorsal tension band is pursued. In any case, the principles from the "superconstruct" concept popularized by Sammarco should be followed closely because a standard internal fixation will almost invariably fail (**Fig. 9**).[40] Nonetheless, there is insufficient evidence to recommend primary reconstruction in acute fore- and/or midfoot fractures in CN with scattered case reports and only one case series of 14 patients with acute stage 1 midfoot CN treated with adequate anatomic reduction and primary arthrodesis with good clinical outcomes 20 years ago.[50] Another more recent case series of 22 patients with CN with 26 feet was reported by Mittlmeier and colleagues to undergo primary reconstruction but only 4 patients had Stage 1 CN while 7 had Stage 2 CN and 11 had Stage 3 CN. Of these 26 feet, only 9 were midfoot CN while 17 feet were hindfoot CN. The authors suggested that although hindfoot CN is less common than midfoot CN, the hindfoot tends to be more unstable and therefore would tend to require surgery compared with the midfoot.[51] Hence, it is in the authors' opinion that there is inadequate evidence to support early fixation/arthrodesis in acute fore- and midfoot fractures in CN unless it is grossly unstable despite casting with presence of ulcers or impending ulceration.[54] Independent of the primary treatment, a close control of both the local conditions at the foot and the systemic metabolic parameters with adequate, prolonged immobilization and offloading are of utmost importance in treating these difficult medical conditions.

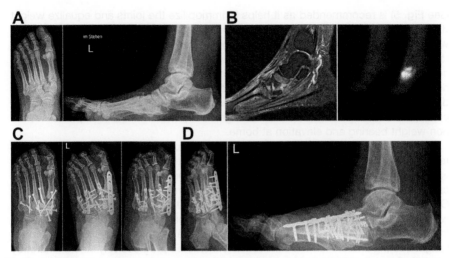

Fig. 9. (*A*) A 67-year-old woman presents with progressive pain, instability, and deformity in her left foot due to CN (Sanders & Frykberg Type II, Brodsky Type 1) for 4 years, aggravated by recent minor trauma. (*B*) MRI revealed extensile bone marrow edema at the midfoot and a Technetium bone scan showed increased uptake at the mid-tarsal and tarsometatarsal joints. (*C*) The initial attempt on primary fusion with screws and one small dorsal plate failed. The patient underwent extensive fixation with small-fragment, variable angle plates. (*D*) At 2-years follow-up, the patient walks in an orthopedic shoe. The left foot is stable, plantigrade, and without ulceration despite complete arch collapse.

RESULTS OF TREATMENT

To the best of our knowledge, there are no clinical studies dealing explicitly with acute mid- and forefoot fractures in diabetics in the absence of CN. In a study of 322 patients, the treatment results of metatarsal fractures were negatively affected by diabetes, BMI, and female sex.[55] Baumfeld and colleagues, when looking at the results of anterograde percutaneous intramedullary fixation for the treatment of lesser metatarsal shaft and neck fractures, found inferior results in women patients with diabetes.[56] The mere presence of diabetes does not seem to affect the generally favorable results after toe fractures.[57]

When comparing 33 patients with diabetes undergoing midfoot, hindfoot, and/or ankle surgery with circular ring fixation to 23 patients with nondiabetics, Wukich and colleagues found a 7-fold risk of complications in the diabetic group and significantly more complications in men.[58]

In contrast, there are several studies on outcomes after operative and nonoperative treatment of midfoot CN.[52] Sinacore, in his classical investigation, found a 100% healing rate of acute (Charcot) fractures, subluxations, or dislocations at an average of 86 ± 45 days by TCC.[59] Acute Charcot arthropathies of the forefoot took less time to heal than those localized to the ankle, hindfoot, or midfoot. Open fractures are prone to soft tissue infection and osteomyelitis.[46]

SUMMARY

The treatment of foot fractures in patients with diabetes is challenging and fraught with complications especially in those with poorly controlled diabetes and CN due to the presence of neuropathy, vasculopathy, and various other medical comorbidities. Despite the lack of guiding literature for acute fore- and midfoot fractures in patients with diabetes, similarities in treatment principles and strategies have been provided with adaptations from diabetic ankle and hindfoot fractures.

The treatment of acute mid- and forefoot fractures in compliant patients with well-controlled diabetes can be similar to a healthy patient with regular perioperative monitoring. On the other hand, patients with poorly controlled diabetes with little or no compliance should be treated with extra-precautions. Medical optimization is pursued by a multidisciplinary team and perioperative blood glucose levels should be kept within the normal range to reduce risks of soft tissue and bony complications. Nonoperative management can be considered primarily as most midfoot fractures are more stable when compared with ankle or hindfoot fractures if there is no skin tenting with impending ulceration or pressure ulceration. A staged surgery can be performed later electively for arthrodesis after partial bony consolidation with less extensile approaches. If surgery is necessary acutely, minimally invasive techniques with mini-open or percutaneous incisions are recommended with fixation beyond the fracture site into adjacent stable joints using the strongest fixation devices such as intramedullary bolts and augmented fixation with transarticular pinning, external fixation, or MIPO bridge plating ("superconstructs"). Prolonged immobilization and non-weight bearing for 8 to 12 weeks are necessary.

In terms of acute foot fractures in CN, the mainstay of treatment should be prolonged immobilization and non-weight bearing in a well-padded cast followed by TCC to allow consolidation. Primary surgical reconstruction during acute stage 1 of CN is controversial. Stabilization with superconstructs is indicated if there is gross instability with impending ulceration or pressure ulceration. Regardless of the choice of treatment, prolonged offloading and immobilization followed by lifelong professional foot care and diabetes management is crucial.

CLINICS CARE POINTS

- In the absence of clinical studies on that topic, the following recommendations about the management of acute and subacute fractures and dislocations at the fore- and midfoot in patients with diabetes reflect the authors' experience and conclusions drawn from the treatment of ankle and hindfoot fractures in diabetics:

- In compliant patients with *good diabetic control* as evident by the HbA1c and blood glucose level trends, indications to surgery and after treatment can be similar to patients without diabetes.

- In patients with *poorly controlled diabetes* and questionable compliance with acute fractures, extreme caution with medical optimization should be exercised whether it is treated operatively or nonoperatively. Stable internal fixation in case of surgical treatment and prolonged offloading independent of the choice of treatment is the mainstay of management in these patients.

- In the presence of *manifest CN*, standard internal fixation and after treatment will invariably fail. The main goals of treatment are to achieve a plantigrade, stable foot that is free of infection and ulceration, and ambulant with orthopedic shoes. Operative treatment is mainly chosen for gross instability or deformity leading to ulceration or inability to walk. In these cases, the concept of fixation with superconstructs in combination with prolonged protection in a well-padded TCC is applied.

- Irrespective of the kind of treatment, tight control of blood glucose levels and other important metabolic parameters is crucial for success.

DISCLOSURE

Stefan Rammelt is a paid consultant for KLS Martin and 3M. He receives travel support from AO Trauma. No conflits of interest result for the purpose of this review.

REFERENCES

1. Beaglehole R, Bonita R, Horton R, et al, Lancet NCD Action Group, NCD Alliance. Priority actions for the non-communicable disease crisis. Lancet 2011;377(9775): 1438–47.
2. Saeedi P, Petersohn I, Salpea P, et al, IDF Diabetes Atlas Committee. Global and regional diabetes prevalence estimates for 2019 and projections for 2030 and 2045: Results from the International Diabetes Federation Diabetes Atlas, 9th edition. Diabetes Res Clin Pract 2019;157:107843.
3. Bommer C, Sagalova V, Heesemann E, et al. Global economic burden of diabetes in adults: projections from 2015 to 2030. Diabetes Care 2018;41(5):963–70.
4. Regan DK, Manoli A 3rd, Hutzler L, et al. Impact of diabetes mellitus on surgical quality measures after ankle fracture surgery: implications for "value-based" compensation and "pay for performance. J Orthop Trauma 2015;29(12):e483–6.
5. Liu JW, Ahn J, Raspovic KM, et al. Increased rates of readmission, reoperation, and mortality following open reduction and internal fixation of ankle fractures are associated with diabetes mellitus. J Foot Ankle Surg 2019;58(3):470–4.
6. Jupiter DC, Hsu ES, Liu GT, et al. Risk factors for short-term complication after open reduction and internal fixation of ankle fractures: analysis of a large insurance claims database. J Foot Ankle Surg 2020;59(2):239–45.
7. Schmidt T, Simske NM, Audet MA, et al. Effects of diabetes mellitus on functional outcomes and complications after torsional ankle fracture. J Am Acad Orthop Surg 2020;28(16):661–70.
8. Cavo MJ, Fox JP, Markert R, et al. Association between diabetes, obesity, and short-term outcomes among patients surgically treated for ankle fracture. J Bone Joint Surg Am 2015;97(12):987–94.
9. Ganesh SP, Pietrobon R, Cecílio WA, et al. The impact of diabetes on patient outcomes after ankle fracture. J Bone Joint Surg Am 2005;87(8):1712–8.
10. Stumpf U, Hadji P, van den Boom L, et al. Incidence of fractures in patients with type 1 diabetes mellitus-a retrospective study with 4420 patients. Osteoporos Int 2020;31(7):1315–22.
11. Wukich DK, Armstrong DG, Attinger CE, et al. Inpatient management of diabetic foot disorders: a clinical guide. Diabetes Care 2013;36(9):2862–71.
12. Rammelt S. Management of acute hindfoot fractures in diabetics. In: Herscovici D Jr, editor. The surgical management of the diabetic foot and ankle: surgical management. Basel, Switzerland: Springer International Publishing; 2016. p. 85–102.
13. Jones KB, Maiers-Yelden KA, Marsh JL, et al. Ankle fractures in patients with diabetes mellitus. J Bone Joint Surg Br 2005;87(4):489–95.
14. Bibbo C, Lin SS, Beam HA, et al. Complications of ankle fractures in diabetic patients. Orthop Clin North Am 2001;32(1):113–33.
15. Gougoulias N, Oshba H, Dimitroulias A, et al. Ankle fractures in diabetic patients. EFORT Open Rev 2020;5(8):457–63.
16. Gandhi A, Liporace F, Azad V, et al. Diabetic fracture healing. Foot Ankle Clin 2006;11(4):805–24.
17. Varma AK. Charcot neuroarthropathy of the foot and ankle: a review. J Foot Ankle Surg 2013;52(6):740–9.

18. Doorgakant A, Davies MB. An approach to managing midfoot charcot deformities. Foot Ankle Clin 2020;25(2):319–35.
19. Thomas R. Diabetic foot disease. In: Chou L, editor. Orthopaedic knowledge update 5, foot and ankle. Rosemont (IL): American Academy of Orthopaedic Surgeons; 2014. p. 67–83.
20. Guyer AJ. Foot and ankle surgery in the diabetic population. Orthop Clin North Am 2018;49(3):381–7.
21. Wukich DK, Sung W. Charcot arthropathy of the foot and ankle: modern concepts and management review. J Diabetes Complications 2009;23(6):409–26.
22. Armstrong DG, Lavery LA, Harkless LB. Who is at risk for diabetic foot ulceration? Clin Podiatr Med Surg 1998;15:11–9.
23. Sohn MW, Stuck RM, Pinzur M, et al. Lower-extremity amputation risk after charcot arthropathy and diabetic foot ulcer. Diabetes Care 2010;33(1):98–100.
24. Frykberg RG, Belczyk R. Epidemiology of the Charcot foot. Clin Podiatr Med Surg 2008;25(1):17–28, v.
25. Wukich DK, Crim BE, Frykberg RG, et al. Neuropathy and poorly controlled diabetes increase the rate of surgical site infection after foot and ankle surgery. J Bone Joint Surg Am 2014;96(10):832–9.
26. Shibuya N, Humphers JM, Fluhman BL, et al. Factors associated with nonunion, delayed union, and malunion in foot and ankle surgery in diabetic patients. J Foot Ankle Surg 2013;52(2):207–11.
27. Qaseem A, Humphrey LL, Chou R, et al. Clinical Guidelines Committee of the American College of Physicians. Use of intensive insulin therapy for the management of glycemic control in hospitalized patients: a clinical practice guideline from the American College of Physicians. Ann Intern Med 2011;154(4):260–7.
28. Moghissi ES, Korytkowski MT, DiNardo M, et al. American Association of Clinical Endocrinologists and American Diabetes Association consensus statement on inpatient glycemic control. Diabetes Care 2009;32(6):1119–31.
29. Ishikawa S. Diabetic foot. In: Canale S, Beaty J, editors. Campbell's operative orthopaedics. 12th edition. Philadelphia (PA): Elsevier Mosby; 2013. p. 4057–77.
30. Heidari N, Charalambous A, Kwok I, et al. Does revascularization prior to foot and ankle surgery reduce the incidence of surgical site infection (SSI)? Foot Ankle Int 2019;40(1_suppl):15S–6S.
31. Althoff A, Cancienne JM, Cooper MT, et al. Patient-related risk factors for periprosthetic ankle joint infection: an analysis of 6977 total ankle arthroplasties. J Foot Ankle Surg 2018;57(2):269–72.
32. Myers TG, Lowery NJ, Frykberg RG, et al. Ankle and hindfoot fusions: comparison of outcomes in patients with and without diabetes. Foot Ankle Int 2012; 33(1):20–8.
33. Rammelt S, Swords M, Dhillon M, et al. Manual of Fracture Management Foot and ankle. Thieme, Stuttgart (Germany), New York and AO: Foundation, Davos (Switzerland); 2020.
34. Anderson BM, Wise BT, Joshi M, et al. Admission hyperglycemia is a risk factor for deep surgical-site infection in orthopaedic trauma patients. J Orthop Trauma 2021;35(12):e451–7.
35. Flynn JM, Rodriguez-del Rio F, Pizá PA. Closed ankle fractures in the diabetic patient. Foot Ankle Int 2000;21(4):311–9.
36. Lovy AJ, Dowdell J, Keswani A, et al. Nonoperative versus operative treatment of displaced ankle fractures in diabetics. Foot Ankle Int 2017;38(3):255–60.
37. Chou LB, Lee DC. Current concept review: perioperative soft tissue management for foot and ankle fractures. Foot Ankle Int 2009;30(1):84–90.

38. Sirkin M, Sanders R, DiPasquale T, et al. A staged protocol for soft tissue management in the treatment of complex pilon fractures. J Orthop Trauma 1999; 13(2):78–84.

39. Duckworth AD, Jefferies JG, Clement ND, et al. Type C tibial pilon fractures: short- and long-term outcome following operative intervention. Bone Joint J 2016;98-B(8):1106–11.

40. Sammarco VJ. Superconstructs in the treatment of charcot foot deformity: plantar plating, locked plating, and axial screw fixation. Foot Ankle Clin 2009;14(3): 393–407.

41. Rammelt S, Zwipp H. Revision of failed midfoot arthrodesis in Charcot arthropathy. 26th AOFAS Summer Meeting, National Harbor, MD, USA, July 7-10, 2010, Proceedings, pp. 104-106.

42. Jeffcoate W. The causes of the Charcot syndrome. Clin Podiatr Med Surg 2008; 25(1):29–42, vi.

43. Rogers LC, Frykberg RG, Armstrong DG, et al. The Charcot foot in diabetes. Diabetes Care 2011;34(9):2123–9.

44. Jeffcoate WJ, Game F, Cavanagh PR. The role of proinflammatory cytokines in the cause of neuropathic osteoarthropathy (acute Charcot foot) in diabetes. Lancet 2005;366(9502):2058–61.

45. Christensen TM, Simonsen L, Holstein PE, et al. Sympathetic neuropathy in diabetes mellitus patients does not elicit Charcot osteoarthropathy. J Diabetes Complications 2011;25(5):320–4.

46. Holmes GB Jr, Hill N. Fractures and dislocations of the foot and ankle in diabetics associated with Charcot joint changes. Foot Ankle Int 1994;15(4):182–5.

47. Brodsky JW. The diabetic foot. In: Mann RA, Coughlin MJ, editors. Surgery of the foot and ankle. St. Louis (MO): Mosby; 1993.

48. Herbst SA, Jones KB, Saltzman CL. Pattern of diabetic neuropathic arthropathy associated with the peripheral bone mineral density. J Bone Joint Surg Br 2004;86(3):378–83.

49. Schade VL, Andersen CA. A literature-based guide to the conservative and surgical management of the acute Charcot foot and ankle. Diabet Foot Ankle 2015;6: 26627.

50. Simon SR, Tejwani SG, Wilson DL, et al. Arthrodesis as an early alternative to nonoperative management of charcot arthropathy of the diabetic foot. J Bone Joint Surg Am 2000;82-A(7):939–50.

51. Mittlmeier T, Klaue K, Haar P, et al. Should one consider primary surgical reconstruction in charcot arthropathy of the feet? Clin Orthop Relat Res 2010;468(4): 1002–11.

52. Schneekloth BJ, Lowery NJ, Wukich DK. Charcot neuroarthropathy in patients with diabetes: an updated systematic review of surgical management. J Foot Ankle Surg 2016;55(3):586–90.

53. Richter M, Mittlmeier T, Rammelt S, et al. Intramedullary fixation in severe Charcot osteo-neuroarthropathy with foot deformity results in adequate correction without loss of correction - results from a multi-centre study. Foot Ankle Surg 2015;21(4): 269–76.

54. Rammelt S, Zwipp H, Schneiders W. Treatment strategies for Charcot osteoarthropathy. Osteologie 2014;23:107–16 [German].

55. Cakir H, Van Vliet-Koppert ST, Van Lieshout EM, et al. Demographics and outcome of metatarsal fractures. Arch Orthop Trauma Surg 2011;131(2):241–5.

56. Baumfeld D, Macedo BD, Nery C, et al. Anterograde percutaneous treatment of lesser metatarsal fractures: technical description and clinical results. Rev Bras Ortop 2015;47(6):760–4.
57. Van Vliet-Koppert ST, Cakir H, Van Lieshout EM, et al. Demographics and functional outcome of toe fractures. J Foot Ankle Surg 2011;50(3):307–10.
58. Wukich DK, Belczyk RJ, Burns PR, et al. Complications encountered with circular ring fixation in persons with diabetes mellitus. Foot Ankle Int 2008;29(10): 994–1000.
59. Sinacore DR. Acute Charcot arthropathy in patients with diabetes mellitus: healing times by foot location. J Diabetes Complications 1998;12(5):287–93.

Managing Acute Ankle and Hindfoot Fracture in Diabetic Patients

Ngwe Phyo, FRCS (Trauma and Ortho)*,
Alexander Wee, FRCS (Trauma and Ortho)

KEYWORDS

• Ankle fracture • Hindfoot fracture • Diabetic neuropathy • Charcot neuroarthropathy

KEY POINTS

• Diabetic patients with ankle fracture risk a higher incidence of complication after injury and treatment.
• Understanding of pathophysiology relating to undesired outcomes is crucial.
• Caution is required when nonoperative management is considered for ankle fracture in patients with peripheral neuropathy.
• Limb salvage should be the key objective.

INTRODUCTION

Diabetes is a growing global problem; the World Health Organization reports that approximately 422 million people worldwide are affected. The prevalence of type 2 adult-onset disease is rising, affecting countries in the developed and developing world.[1] The impact of the disease has been mitigated with technology, modern therapies, and medication, allowing patients with the condition to maintain their functional status.

Ankle fractures are one of the commonest injuries presented at emergency departments. Hindfoot fractures such as talus and calcaneal fractures are less common. According to recent reports, the incidence of diabetes in patients with ankle fractures ranges from 1 in 20 to as high as 1 in 7. Ganesh and colleagues[2] in 2005 undertook a nationwide retrospective study of surgically treated ankle fractures in the United States, which showed 5.71% of their 160,000 patients suffered from diabetes. More recently, Schmidt and colleagues[3] retrospectively reviewed a cohort of nearly 1000 patients with surgically managed ankle fracture in their center, over 13-year period, and found that 13.4% of the patient population had diabetes.

Department of Trauma and Orthopaedics, Frimley Park Hospital, Frimley Health NHS Foundation Trust, Portsmouth Road, Camberley GU16 7UJ, UK
* Corresponding author.
E-mail address: ngwe.phyo@nhs.net

Foot Ankle Clin N Am 27 (2022) 639–654
https://doi.org/10.1016/j.fcl.2022.02.002
1083-7515/22/Crown Copyright © 2022 Published by Elsevier Inc. All rights reserved.

Reviews of diabetic patients with ankle fractures have demonstrated a higher incidence of complications after injury and treatment. Outcome measures and complications such as length of hospital stay, reoperation rate, wound breakdown, surgical site infection, nonunion, and Charcot neuroarthropathy are significantly higher in this group of patients.[2–5]

There is a canon of work recording poor patient outcomes in diabetic patients with ankle fractures, with the consensus that management of these injuries requires careful deliberation. At the same time, this predicament has swayed risk-averse surgeons to regard nonoperative treatment as a "safer" alternative.[6] However, there is evidence demonstrating ankle fractures treated nonoperatively in diabetic patients result in suboptimal outcomes, convincing fracture surgeons to offer surgical fixation to maximize the chance of healing.[7]

In this review, the current evidence for the treatment of ankle and hindfoot fractures in diabetic patients is examined. The pathophysiology of diabetes and Charcot neuroarthropathy relevant to ankle and hindfoot fractures and their effects are reviewed and how these might influence treatment is discussed.

PATHOPHYSIOLOGY

Diabetes mellitus affects wound healing, inflammation, vascular inflow, and can lead to Charcot arthropathy. It is therefore important to understand how the condition affects bone biology and fracture healing.

Diabetes is a metabolic disorder characterized by chronic hyperglycemia; an abnormally elevated state of blood sugar concentration, resulting from defects in insulin secretion and resistance to insulin action or both.[8] The clinical criteria for the diagnosis of diabetes include polyuria, polydipsia, unexplained weight loss with one or more of the following tests results: a random blood glucose concentration $\geq$ 11.1 mmol/L ($\geq$200 mg/dL), a fasting plasma glucose concentration $\geq$ 7.0 mmol/L ($\geq$126 mg/dL) measured on 2 separate occasions, a 2-hour plasma glucose concentration greater than 200 mg/dL during following an oral glucose tolerance test and a glycated hemoglobin (HbA1c) level greater than 48 mmol/mol (6.5%).[9]

Two distinct forms of diabetes exist: type 1 (5%–10%) is an autoimmune condition in which T lymphocytes cause the destruction of insulin-secreting β-cells in the islets of Langerhans of the pancreas, resulting in a state of insulin deficiency. Type 2 (90%–95%)[10] is a complex condition resulting from insulin insensitivity in peripheral tissue, along with β-cell dysfunction causing inadequate insulin output. The effect of chronic hyperglycemia on body organ systems is widespread. Damage to small- and medium-sized arteries gives rise to disruption of blood supply to target organs, especially in areas such as the peripheral nerves, kidneys, retina, and so forth. The development of tissue injury in major organ system leads to well-defined clinical states such as peripheral neuropathy, nephropathy, retinopathy, peripheral vascular disease, hypertension, and so forth. In addition to these, people with diabetes show increased susceptibility to infection due to a hyperglycemic tissue environment that nurtures poor host defenses while enduring impaired oxygen delivery as a result of microangiopathy and macroangiopathy.[11] Furthermore, wound healing potential is hindered due to local ischemia and elevated blood glucose level. Local tissue oxygen tension influences collagen synthesis and deposition in fractures and wounds. Collagen produced in a low oxygen environment may not have the ability to contribute to optimal wound strength.[12]

Slow fracture healing in patients with diabetes is well recognized. Macey and colleagues[13] found that reduced collagen synthesis causes diminished tensile strength and stiffness of healing callus in their animal model. Similarly, another animal study reported that diabetic mice produce a sufficient amount of immature mesenchymal tissue but fail to adequately express genes that regulate osteoblast differentiation, which, in turn, leads to decreased bone formation.[14]

One of the common complications of diabetes is peripheral neuropathy affecting 50% of all diabetics. Protective and proprioceptive sensations in the lower limbs are affected; patients are unaware of injury to the extremity. This makes them vulnerable to ulceration and, more likely to neglect trauma. The absence of protective sensation in patients with diabetes has been recognized as the key symptom that is predictive of the potential for the development of Charcot neuroarthropathy.[15]

Two distinct theories have been proposed as to the potential etiology of Charcot arthropathy: the neurotraumatic and neurovascular theory. The neurotraumatic theory postulates that an initial injury, either a single event or repetitive microtrauma, triggers the process of bony destruction. Continued loading of the foot leads to eventual structural failure, followed by a healing process. The neurovascular theory proposes an autonomic neuropathy causes a hyperdynamic blood flow with arteriovenous shunting. This results in osteoclastic stimulation, increased bone turnover, and local osteopenia—predisposing the bone to fracture and the foot to collapse. Proinflammatory mediators are believed to take part in this process: acute Charcot is an inflammatory response to an initiating traumatic event, mediated through the increased expression of proinflammatory cytokines, including tumor necrosis factor α (TNFα) and interleukin 1β. This acute-phase inflammatory process is also responsible for the healing process in fracture, facilitating the lysis of fracture fragments, leading to new bone formation. TNFα and interleukin 1β together initiate increased expression of receptor activator nuclear transcription factor κB (NF-κB) ligand (RANKL), causing osteoclast maturation and promoting osteolysis in the area.[16] An injury to the ankle or hindfoot in diabetic patients with neuropathy is sufficient to trigger this exaggerated inflammatory process. The combined effects of an amplified inflammatory response, impaired collagen and bone synthesis, vasculopathy and neuropathy profoundly affects the outcome of ankle and hindfoot fractures.

ANKLE FRACTURE
Clinical Assessment

The importance of a thorough review of a patient's background medical history and assessment of clinical features in ankle fracture patients with diabetes cannot be overemphasized. Long-term glycemic control, renal and vascular function, preinjury mobility, and previous ulceration and infection are important factors of the patient interview. The history of trauma should focus on the mechanism of injury, the energy involved, and if there was any mobility after injury and delay in presentation. Scrutiny of available past medical history is advantageous and often assists formulation of a treatment plan.

A thorough clinical examination is vital. Signs of soft tissue contusion, swelling, limb posture, presence of erythema, skin integrity, and pedal pulses allude to the severity of the injury. Assessment of peripheral neuropathy and protective sensation is commonly omitted in the acute trauma setting. Foot sensation should be assessed ideally with Semmes-Weinstein monofilament before plaster slab for immobilization is applied. Alternatively, it can be assessed in between plaster changes. However, it could be argued that test reliability may be affected by the patient's general discomfort after injury, and their state of anxiety after ankle fracture. Practically, one could consider performing the test on the contralateral limb and use the results in general, as lower limb peripheral neuropathy affects both sides more or less equally.[17]

Assessment of foot circulation is carried out by examining both anterior and posterior tibial artery pulses. A handheld Doppler ultrasound probes provide additional information on the sonographic characteristics of the arterial waveform, which is an indicator of the degree of arteriosclerosis. Another noninvasive assessment of peripheral arterial disease is the Ankle Brachial Pressure Index (ABPI): calculated as the ratio between systolic blood pressure at the level of ankle to that of the brachial artery. An ABPI of less than 0.9 suggests peripheral vascular disease. In the authors' center, ABPI is not routinely performed in ankle fracture patients with diabetes because of impracticalities associated with ankle swelling, pain, and cast immobilization. A transcutaneous oxygen pressure (T_cPO_2) measurement is routinely performed—a value of 30 mm Hg or less indicates poor tissue oxygenation and is a predictive factor for poor wound healing.[18] Early discussion with the vascular service is necessary if there are significant features of limb ischemia, which may potentially require revascularization.

Patients with complicated diabetes—neuropathy, nephropathy, vasculopathy, retinopathy, and poor glycemic control—have a greater risk of poorer functional outcomes after ankle fractures.[5] A multidisciplinary diabetic team approach is advocated, as the management of such medical complications is beyond the remit of trauma and orthopedic surgeons, especially in patients with complex diabetes. An HbA1c level of more than 6.5% (69 mmol/mol Hb), indicating poor diabetic control, is a risk factor for poor outcome in diabetic patients with an ankle fracture.[19] In patients with a chronic renal disease requiring regular dialysis, HbA1c level might not reflect accurate glycemic status because of shortened erythrocyte life span. In this scenario, glycated albumin or fructosamine level can be used as an alternative.[20,21] These patients need to be assessed by an endocrinologist for optimization of their perioperative glycemic control, thereby lowering the risk of perioperative and postoperative complications. It is therefore imperative that the treating surgeon, right from the outset, has a candid discussion with such patients about the potential for poor outcomes and complications after such injuries.

NONOPERATIVE MANAGEMENT

Despite the known association with poorer outcomes, nonoperative treatment is not completely redundant. It has a role in the management of undisplaced or stable ankle fracture patterns, especially in patients with uncomplicated diabetes. Treatment consists of closed contact casting and weight-bearing restriction until fracture healing is demonstrated (**Fig. 1**). This treatment demands close observation and serial radiological assessment, especially in the early treatment period, to monitor skin and soft tissue integrity and capture signs of subtle displacement. Patient compliance is crucial with this strategy. The treating surgeon should also be ready to switch to an alternative treatment strategy when encountering early complications indicating impending failure of nonoperative management.

Schon and colleagues[22] in 1998 reported the results of 32 diabetic neuropathic patients with ankle fractures. Sixteen patients with nondisplaced ankle fractures in the study underwent nonoperative treatment. Three patients were untreated for the initial 6 to 12 weeks, before presenting to the author's institution; they were casted for less than 3 months, resulting in stable, well-aligned ankle, without developing Charcot neuroarthropathy. Five patients had a cast or brace applied for 2 to 3 months with a non–weight-bearing period of up to 6 months, again resulting in stable, well-aligned ankles without Charcot neuroarthropathy. Seven patients had a longer duration of casting for 3 to 9 months with non–weight-bearing maintained for 1 to 4 months, resulting in similar stable, well-aligned ankles. Only 1 patient in this group with a nondisplaced

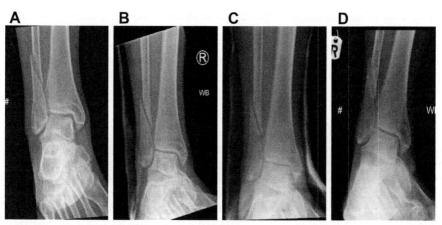

Fig. 1. Lateral malleolus ankle fracture in 55-year-old male diabetic patient with peripheral neuropathy and complex medical comorbidities treated nonoperatively, demonstrating slow union. AP radiography at the time of injury (A), at 3 months (B), at 4 months (C), and at 6 months (D).

Pilon fracture developed a Charcot process but was successfully managed using a total contact cast for 9 months. A total of 16 displaced ankle fractures were included in their study. The treatment journey they reported in 4 displaced ankle fracture patients in this group was compelling. These 4 patients underwent closed reduction and casting initially for 3 months. Owing to noncompliance with weight-bearing restrictions, the initial reduction was lost in 3 patients, leading to surgical intervention. The remaining 1 patient went into a valgus deformity after developing Charcot neuroarthropathy requiring a subsequent ankle arthrodesis. Nine patients underwent open reduction and internal fixation as the initial procedure after acute injury. Three of these 9 patients experienced progressive loss in alignment, despite internal fixation, subsequently requiring hindfoot fusion. The remaining 3 in this group had Pilon fractures requiring a hindfoot intramedullary fusion rod or, a combination of limited internal fixation with hybrid external fixation, so as to achieve a painless stable hindfoot.[22] The article suggests there is a role for nonoperative treatment in undisplaced ankle fractures, although the attending surgeon needs to be vigilant for early displacement, and be prepared to surgically intervene if there are complications. A high level of caution should be exercised when a nonoperative approach is considered for displaced and/or unstable fracture patterns. Loss of reduction and progressive deterioration can often lead to unsatisfactory outcomes, as reported by Schon in their displaced fracture patient group.

In another contemporary study, McCormack and colleagues presented a contrary argument in their report. Based on their findings in a retrospective case-controlled study, it may be preferable to accept a loss of reduction and malunion, instead of risking potential complications, such as deep infection, failure of fixation, wound breakdown, and amputation, which are associated with operative treatment.[6]

More recently in 2017, Lovy and colleagues[7] retrospectively reviewed the outcome of 28 adult diabetic patients with displaced ankle fractures in their center. They found as much as 21-fold increased odds (ratio) of complications in their 20 nonoperatively (closed reduction and casting) treated patients compared with 8 patients who underwent surgical fixation within 3 weeks of injury. As would be expected, loss of reduction was the most common complication (55%), followed by new-onset Charcot neuroarthropathy (35%), ulceration (25%), unplanned surgery (25%), and deep infection

(10%). They noted that loss of reduction occurred within the first 6 weeks after injury. Seven patients in their cohort developed Charcot changes, as early as 8 weeks after injury, 4 requiring arthrodesis. Furthermore, the complication rate following unplanned surgical fixation in the presence of persistent nonunion or malunion in nonoperatively treated patients was 100% compared with 12.5% in the immediate planned fixation group.

OPERATIVE MANAGEMENT

Standard surgical management of displaced ankle fractures requires open reduction and internal fixation of displaced fragments using established osteosynthesis principles and techniques. The procedure requires atraumatic soft tissue handling, anatomic reduction of the articular surfaces, stable fixation of the intraarticular fragments, and use of appropriate hardware for construct stability. After surgical fixation, early active motion is encouraged to maximize the potential for functional recovery. Although these principles provide a framework for planning surgical treatment for ankle fractures in complex diabetics, this group of physiologically compromised patients merits extra consideration and attention to implant choice and fixation techniques.

Initial management must include elevating the injured limb on a Braun-Bohler frame or pillows to allow the swelling to reduce. The injury edema should be monitored by clinical assessment so that surgery can be timed for when the soft tissues allow. In highly unstable fractures, loss of reduction can occur despite the plaster backslab, this is often the cause of swelling and deformity that fails to improve with elevation and rest. When in doubt, prompt assessment of fracture position using appropriate imaging is imperative. An external fixator can be used to maintain fracture reduction while allowing soft tissue swelling to resolve before definitive surgical fixation can take place. A period of 7 to 10 days is typically required before postinjury swelling settles to a level that allows surgical treatment. This is heralded by the reduction of skin turgor and the appearance of skin wrinkles over the planned surgical incision sites.

Standard ankle fracture fixation technique with small fragment hardware—one-third tubular plating and medial 4.5 mm screws—is inadequate in patients with complex diabetes, as the risk of Charcot neuroarthropathy and failure of fixation in the pathologic bone is high. Costigan and colleagues[23] reported 14% complication rate in their large retrospective case series (12 of 84 patients) of operatively managed ankle fracture in patients with diabetes. The average age of the patient was 49 years and followup was 4 years. They used standard fixation techniques with small fragment hardware in all their patients. Weight-bearing commenced in cast at 4 to 8 weeks after surgery. Nine patients in their cohort had an open ankle fracture. Their infection rate was 13% (10 in 84), with 8 patients needing further surgery including 2 subsequent transtibial amputations. Only 4 patients in their group developed Charcot changes. One patient with an open fracture required transtibial amputation following Charcot process. In their analyses, they found no correlation between the type of ankle fracture and complication rate. Similarly, open fracture, insulin dependence, and patient age had no significant effect on outcomes. However, a significantly increased risk of complication was noted in patients with peripheral neuropathy or absent pedal pulses.[23]

As early as 1995, the risk of fixation failure in complex diabetics was recognized, prompting Schon to advocate the use of multiple tetracortical syndesmotic screw fixation to augment stability of the hardware construct (**Fig. 2**). This was combined with an extended period of immobilization and protected weight-bearing.[24] Dunn later corroborated this by testing augmented fixation of the distal fibula in cadavers. He

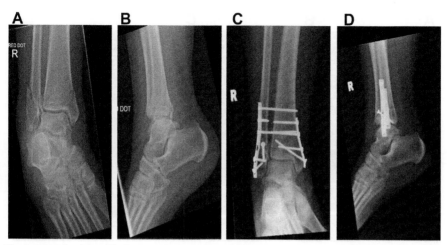

Fig. 2. Bimalleolar ankle fracture in a 45-year-old female insulin-dependent diabetic patient with peripheral neuropathy (*A, B*), after operative treatment using tetracortical fibula to tibia fixation (*C, D*).

demonstrated improved mean stiffness and strength to failure with axial loading when compared with plate fixation with intramedullary Kirschner wires.[25] Perry and colleagues used the same technique but with a 4.5 mm dynamic compression plate and multiple 4.5 mm tetracortical syndesmotic screws instead of the traditional one-third tubular plate, for salvage fixation in 6 failed neuropathic ankle fracture patients. The author reported all 6 patients were satisfied with their results, averting the prospect of below knee amputation.[26] This technique of fixing the syndesmosis with multiple screws raises concerns of altering gait and the biomechanics of walking unfavorably. However, progressive mobilization restores motion between tibia and fibula despite the presence of syndesmotic screws.[27]

A retrospective case-control study conducted by Wukich and colleagues[5] in 2011 looked at the complications of ankle fracture in patients with complicated versus uncomplicated diabetes. Unsurprisingly, patients with complicated diabetes had 3.8 times increased risk of overall complication, 3.4 times risk of noninfectious complication (malunion, nonunion, or Charcot neuroarthropathy), and 5 times risk of revision surgery when compared with patients with uncomplicated diabetes. They also looked at different surgical fixation methods used to treat ankle fractures. Types of surgical fixation were grouped into (1) standard open reduction internal fixation (ORIF) using distal fibula plate and lag screw, (2) similar fixation of distal fibula and with 2 or more tetracortical tibiofibular screws and/or transarticular pin fixation, coining the term ORIF Plus, (3) both internal and external fixation, and (4) external fixation alone. The authors found that patients who had ORIF Plus had significantly fewer overall complications than those treated with other techniques. Higher rates of complication were seen in those patients treated with combined internal and external fixation, and external fixation alone than those treated with standard ORIF and ORIF Plus.[5]

Although preserving motion in the ankle joint would be the ideal outcome, primary ankle arthrodesis may have a role in certain cases where injury to the articular surface is extensive or, overall bony architecture in the ankle area is too deformed to carry out internal fixation (**Fig. 3**). Ayoub reported the result of his case series in which 17 diabetic patients with an unstable ankle fracture complicated by Charcot neuroarthropathy underwent primary ankle fusion as a salvage procedure.[28] The mean age of their cohort

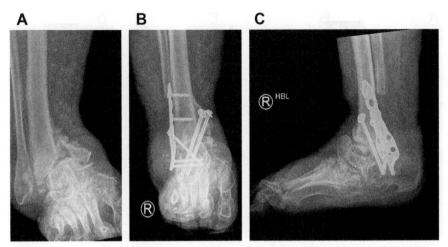

Fig. 3. Charcot neuroarthropathy of the ankle in a 70-year-old female diabetic patient with peripheral neuropathy after nonoperative treatment of unstable ankle fracture (*A*), with subsequent hindfoot arthrodesis using compression screw and plate (*B*, *C*) achieving stable union and good alignment.

was 62 years and follow-up was 26 months. All patients were treated nonoperatively before presenting to the author's institute. Open tibiotalar arthrodesis was carried out using 2 to 3 crossed-screw technique. Autologous bone graft from resected malleoli was used in all cases. The author reported achieving a stable ankle in 14 of 17 patients (82%), 9 bony unions and 5 with stiff fibrous ankylosis. Arthrodesis failed in 3 patients owing to talar avascular necrosis, leading to poor joint stability, subsequent ulceration of soft tissue, and eventually, major amputation. Wallace and colleagues[29] reported the results of ankle arthrodesis in 13 ankle fractures in diabetic patients with peripheral neuropathy. They used circular limb external fixation for patients with open wounds and osteomyelitis, whereas an intramedullary nail was used for those patients with closed fractures or without infection. The group reported a favorable clinical outcome in 11 of 13 patients at a mean follow-up of 48 months (12–136 months) after the initial surgery. Limb salvage was achieved in 12 of 13 patients, 8 with evidence of radiological union, 3 with stable pseudoarthrosis using therapeutic footwear.

Retrograde hindfoot nails have been used to treat ankle fractures in neuropathic patients achieving good results.[30,31] Ebaugh and colleagues reported outcomes of primary hindfoot nailing for complicated diabetic ankle fractures. Their retrospective case series included 27 patients, with a mean age of 66 years (range, 32–92 years) treated with tibiotalocalcaneal nailing for ankle fracture as primary treatment without joint preparation. They reported 96% salvage rate, 88% union rate, with mean time to weight-bearing 6.7 weeks. Authors argued that hindfoot stiffness following retrograde nailing was well tolerated in their study population due to lower functional demands and neuropathic limbs (**Fig. 4**). With high limb salvage rates, low complication rates, and acceptable return to preinjury ambulation, the authors advocated this stabilization technique as a viable option.[31]

Regardless of the type of surgical fixation device used, an important fact to consider when treating ankle fractures in complex neuropathic diabetic patients is their lower functional demands for ambulation. A successful outcome is one that maintains the patient's ambulatory function and avoids a major amputation.

POSTOPERATIVE WEIGHT-BEARING

An extended period of protected weight-bearing in a cast or brace is a common practice for these patients, regardless of treatment strategy, surgical or not. This principle is based on the knowledge that this cohort of patients has slower bone healing and loss of protective sensation. This combination reduces their awareness of early fixation or bone failure (**Fig. 5**). Schon and colleagues[24] advocated prolonged immobilization as one of the key principles in treating these fractures. An extensive period of 6 to 12 months of protected weight-bearing may be necessary, depending on the complexity and severity of the fracture. A similar observation was reported by Wukich and colleagues[15] following review of the evidence in his 2008 article. This concept of prolonged protected weight-bearing was evaluated in a study by Bazarov and colleagues[32] by retrospectively analyzing 73 diabetic patients with a closed ankle fracture. All patients were allowed to start protected weight-bearing in a cast or boot at 2 weeks after injury or surgery. They reported 25% complication rate in the surgery group, with wound dehiscence being most common, and 8% in the nonsurgery group, with different complications such as loss of reduction and mal/nonunion. Despite reporting a 25% complication rate, authors claimed there is evidence to support earlier weight-bearing in carefully selected patients with fewer comorbidities.

Rosenbaum and colleagues in 2013 surveyed a body of American Foot and Ankle surgeons, seeking a consensus of treatment techniques in diabetics with ankle fractures. He found the majority would favor an enhanced fixation method with an extended period of non–weight-bearing of between 8 and 12 weeks for patients with displaced ankle fractures. The survey also indicated that most surgeons would treat undisplaced ankle fractures in a plaster cast.[33]

TALUS FRACTURE

Talus fractures and peritalar dislocations in patients with diabetes need to be managed similar to nondiabetic population. Depending on the type of fracture pattern and

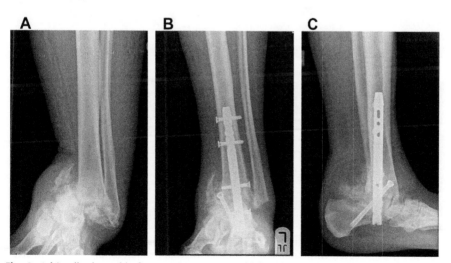

Fig. 4. A bimalleolar ankle fracture in a 65-year-old female patient initially treated nonoperatively leading to loss of reduction and deformity (A), with subsequent tibiotalocalcaneal arthrodesis using a hindfoot nail (B, C) achieving bone union and good alignment.

dislocation involved, appropriate treatment plans need to be devised, taking into consideration of soft tissue envelope, status of peripheral circulation, risk of avascular necrosis, patient's smoking status. The early fragmentation phase in the Charcot neuro-arthropathy process can occasionally mimic the radiological appearance of fracture in the talus. Careful assessment of background information, especially nature of the trauma sustained and presence of peripheral neuropathy, should help the physician reach the correct diagnosis. In these cases, a total contact cast to maintain overall align-ment until Charcot inflammatory process has resolved may be all that is required. Reg-ular cast changes and soft tissue assessment is imperative to monitor the integrity of the skin under threat of ulceration from bony prominence. Tibiotalocalcaneal arthrodesis with an intramedullary device may be necessary in cases where hindfoot instability on weight-bearing threatens the soft tissue integrity. There is no available literature report-ing on the treatment and outcomes of these injuries in diabetic patients.

CALCANEAL FRACTURE

Calcaneal fracture can occur without significant trauma in patients with diabetes. Generally, 3 distinct fracture patterns have been recognised.[34] (1) Bony avulsion of pos-terior calcaneal tuberosity, usually involving the posterior third of the calcaneus with pri-mary fracture line parallel to apophyseal growth plate. It is commonly associated with displacement of superior cortex but without extension to inferior cortex (**Fig. 6**). This type of avulsion injury is considered to be an insufficiency fracture as the pattern is similar in nondiabetic patients as a result of a tight Achilles tendon leading to a failure

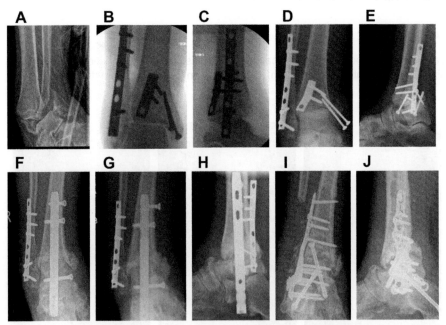

Fig. 5. A trimalleolar ankle fracture in a 66-year-old female diabetic patient with peripheral neuropathy (A), treated with open reduction and internal fixation (B, C), subsequent fixa-tion failure leading to loss of reduction at 2 months after surgery (D, E), revised to tibiota-localcaneal fusion using a hindfoot nail (F), subsequent nonunion and hardware failure (G, H) and revision hindfoot arthrodesis using a plate (I, J).

of the bone in tension.[35] Surgical fixation may only be required in cases where a significant displacement of avulsed fragment has occurred preventing bony union. In small or minimally displaced fractures, nonoperative management with foot in plantar flexion cast would facilitate healing. Malunion secondary to proximal fragment migration does not tend to impact this patient group significantly.[24] (2) Midbody compression type fracture, where the fracture is confined to the body of calcaneus running horizontally parallel to the talocalcaneal joint without breaching the joint surface (**Fig. 7**). Schon advocated conservative treatment for this fracture, especially if there is a concurrent Charcot process.[24] Residual deformity or post-traumatic symptomatic arthritis can be treated with an arthrodesis. (3) Tongue type fractures, in which the fracture line extends from posterior calcaneal tuberosity toward talocalcaneal joint (**Fig. 8**). A degree of superior displacement is commonly observed with this pattern. Surgical fixation may be required to reduce the fragment and to prevent overlying soft tissue necrosis. Diligent monitoring of the skin and soft tissue is advisable if fixation is delayed.

The risk of complications is raised if there is an associated heel ulcer (**Fig. 9**). Patients often report a sudden give or pop in the heel. The combination of a tight Achilles and a weakened calcaneus results in this injury pattern. The ulcer and underlying infected bone require thorough debridement before stabilization of the fracture which facilitates bone healing. To mitigate the strong Achilles pull, transection of the Achilles tendon is a useful technique to bring the displaced fragment down. Instead of using standard screw fixation in the presence of infection, multiple heavy threaded wires can be applied into the calcaneus to hold the reduction. These wires can remain in situ for 8 to 12 months. Following debridement of the ulcer and surrounding soft tissue, the resulting defect is managed using vacuum-assisted closure wound therapy and the patient is kept non–weight-bearing until wires are removed.[36] Plastic surgery with a soft tissue flap may be required in some cases.[37]

Percutaneous wiring or a circular limb external fixator can be used for primary subtalar joint arthrodesis in traumatic calcaneal fracture with multiple comminutions in diabetic patients where soft tissue envelope is not optimal for open surgical techniques.[38]

SUMMARY

Diabetes influences bone healing after injury. There is a well-founded reluctance for treating fractures in these patients for fear of serious complications. Patients with diabetes are not uniform; some have uncomplicated disease, with excellent metabolic control. In this group of patients, fracture management and operative techniques similar to nondiabetics can be used. They usually require an extra degree of postoperative care and vigilance for early complications such as displacement, fixation failure, or development of the Charcot process. Their trajectory of recovery and function is close to that of nondiabetic patients.

Patients with complex diabetes—multiple comorbidities—have a worse risk profile, and it is this group that causes much concern among surgeons. Seemingly straightforward fractures might be the initiation of a Charcot process and, if treated in the same way as a nondiabetic patient, the risk of fracture displacement and progression of the Charcot process is high. Surgeons must have a low index of suspicion for the development of Charcot when assessing the patient and examining for peripheral neuropathy. Patients with chronic limb ischemia need to be identified before surgical fixation. Patients with peripheral vascular disease have a higher risk of wound complications, failure of fixation, and, ultimately, amputation. This group needs assessment and optimization by a vascular surgeon before any orthopedic intervention.

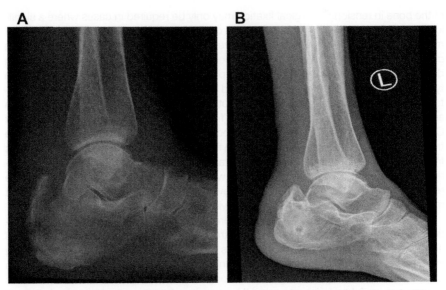

Fig. 6. An avulsion fracture of calcaneal tuberosity (*A*) in a 47-year-old female diabetic patient, treated nonoperatively. Radiological appearance of bony union at 12 months (*B*).

Surgical technique must be carefully considered in this subgroup of patients with complicated diabetes; conventional techniques and hardware may be inadequate. Ankle fractures require more robust fixation, with surgeons electing to use augmented fixation with tetracortical screws, low contour dynamic compression plates, locking plates, or intramedullary nailing techniques. Critics have commented that the dynamics of the gait cycle will be adversely affected, as the ankle is stiffened. Follow-up and functional studies have shown that, in practice, for this group of low demand and low functional activity patients, this has a minimal bearing. The logical progression of this is the role for primary fusion of the ankle and/or hindfoot in these patients.

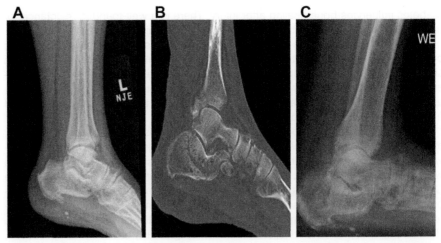

Fig. 7. A midbody compression fracture of calcaneus (*A, B*) in a 78-year-old female diabetic patient, treated nonoperatively. Radiological appearance of bony union at 6 months (*C*).

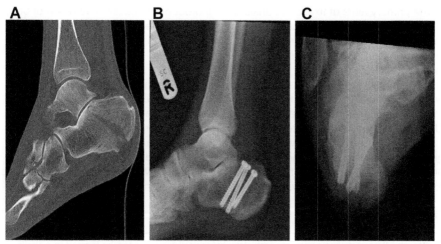

Fig. 8. A tongue-type fracture of calcaneus (*A*), treated with internal fixation (*B*, *C*).

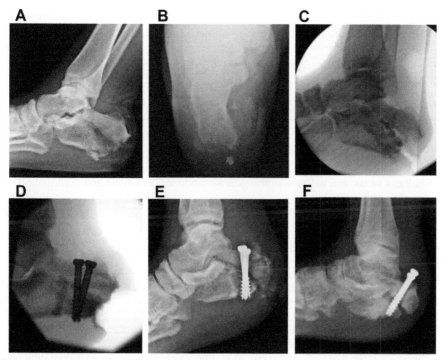

Fig. 9. A calcaneal fracture in a 54-year-old female patient with associated heel ulcer (*A*), an arrow showing osteomyelitis in calcaneal tuberosity (*B*), intraoperative image after initial debridement and application of antibiotic-loaded bone substitute (*C*), a further debridement 2 weeks later and fracture fixation (*D*), radiological appearance of early fixation failure at 3 weeks (*E*), and a stable union of 10 months (*F*). Screws were subsequently removed electively.

The primary aims of fixation of ankle and hindfoot fractures are restoration of bony anatomy, joint realignment, and maintenance of movement. In diabetic patients with multiple comorbidities, the aim is to heal the fracture and preserve the limb; amputation increases the metabolic demands of the patient and lowers their life expectancy significantly.[39]

Diabetes has an effect on osteoblasts and collagen metabolism and, as a result, wound and bone fracture healing are prolonged. The time of immobilization and protected weight-bearing in a cast needs to be reconsidered and lengthened. There is also the concern of disuse osteopenia which can result from prolonged immobilization.

Complex diabetic patients with ankle and hindfoot fractures can be treated with surgery. Their outcomes are poorer than nondiabetics, and the risk of complication is higher. The aim is to achieve fracture healing, maintain a well-aligned limb, be vigilant for Charcot neuroarthropathy, and minimize the risk of amputation.

CLINICS CARE POINTS

- Uncomplicated diabetic patients with straightforward fractures can be treated in a similar way to nondiabetic patients. They require greater vigilance during the treatment period
- Complicated diabetes is not a contraindication to operative management of ankle fractures.
- Critical limb ischemia is a relative contraindication to surgical treatment. These patients need vascular assessment and optimization before fixation.
- Augmented fixation techniques with stronger implants should be used in operative fixation.
- Primary fusion of the ankle and subtalar joint has a role in the treatment of fractures in complex diabetic patients.
- Be vigilant for Charcot neuroarthropathy and be prepared to intervene if necessary.
- Amputation increases the energy requirement for mobilization and reduces life expectancy.
- Patients may require a longer cast immobilization period and protected weight-bearing.

ACKNOWLEDGMENTS

The authors would like to thank Anthony Sakellariou for his advice and contribution in preparation of the article.

DISCLOSURE

The authors have nothing to disclose.

REFERENCES

1. Diabetes. Available at: https://www.who.int/news-room/fact-sheets/detail/diabetes. Accessed May 12, 2020.
2. Ganesh SP, Pietrobon R, Cecílio WA, et al. The impact of diabetes on patient outcomes after ankle fracture. J Bone Joint Surg Am 2005;87(8):1712–8.
3. Schmidt T, Simske NM, Audet MA, et al. Effects of diabetes mellitus on functional outcomes and complications after torsional ankle fracture. J Am Acad Orthop Surg 2020;28(16):661–70.
4. Regan DK, Manoli A, Hutzler L, et al. Impact of diabetes mellitus on surgical quality measures after ankle fracture surgery: implications for "value-based" compensation and "pay for performance. J Orthop Trauma 2015;29(12):e483–6.

5. Wukich DK, Joseph A, Ryan M, et al. Outcomes of ankle fractures in patients with uncomplicated versus complicated diabetes. Foot Ankle Int 2011;32(2):120–30.

6. McCormack RG, Leith JM. Ankle fractures in diabetics. Complications of surgical management. J Bone Joint Surg Br 1998;80(4):689–92.

7. Lovy AJ, Dowdell J, Keswani A, et al. Nonoperative versus operative treatment of displaced ankle fractures in diabetics. Foot Ankle Int 2017;38(3):255–60.

8. World Health Organization. Definition, diagnosis and classification of diabetes mellitus and its complications. Part 1:WHO published report; 1999. doi:WHO/NCD/NCS/99.2 ed

9. Diabetes UK. Diagnostic criteria for diabetes - Diabetes UK. 2016. Available at: https://www.diabetes.org.uk/professionals/position-statements-reports/diagnosis-ongoing-management-monitoring/new_diagnostic_criteria_for_diabetes. Accessed September 6, 2021.

10. Classification of diabetes mellitus 2019 Classification of diabetes mellitus. 2019. Available at: http://apps.who.int/bookorders. Accessed September 6, 2021.

11. Casqueiro J, Casqueiro J, Alves C. Infections in patients with diabetes mellitus: a review of pathogenesis. Indian J Endocrinol Metab 2012;16(Suppl1):S27.

12. Jonsson K, Jensen JA, Goodson WH, et al. Tissue Oxygenation, Anemia, and Perfusion in Relation to Wound Healing in Surgical Patients. Ann Surg 1991; 214(5):603–13.

13. Macey L, Kana S, Jingushi S, et al. Defects of early fracture-healing in experimental diabetes. J Bone Joint Surg Am 1989;71(5):722–33.

14. Lu H, Kraut D, Gerstenfeld LC, et al. Diabetes interferes with the bone formation by affecting the expression of transcription factors that regulate osteoblast differentiation. Endocrinology 2003;144(1):346–52.

15. Wukich DK, Kline AJ. The management of ankle fractures in patients with diabetes. J Bone Joint Surg Am 2008;90(7):1570–8.

16. Jeffcoate W, Game F, Cavanagh P. The role of proinflammatory cytokines in the cause of neuropathic osteoarthropathy (acute Charcot foot) in diabetes. Lancet 2005;366:2058–61.

17. Pasnoor M, Dimachkie MM, Kluding P, et al. Diabetic neuropathy part 1: overview and symmetric phenotypes. 2013. doi:10.1016/j.ncl.2013.02.004

18. Got I. [Transcutaneous oxygen pressure (TcPO2): advantages and limitations]. Diabetes Metab 1998;24(4):379–84.

19. Liu J, Ludwig T, Ebraheim NA. Effect of the blood HbA1c level on surgical treatment outcomes of diabetics with ankle fractures. 2013. doi:10.1111/os.12047

20. Divani M, Georgianos PI, Didangelos T, et al. Comparison of glycemic markers in chronic hemodialysis using continuous glucose monitoring. Am J Nephrol 2018; 47(1):21–9.

21. Bomholt T, Feldt-Rasmussen B, Butt R, et al. Hemoglobin A1c and fructosamine evaluated in patients with type 2 diabetes receiving peritoneal dialysis using long-term continuous glucose monitoring. Nephron 2022;146:146–52.

22. Schon LC, Easley ME, Weinfeld SB. Charcot neuroarthropathy of the foot and ankle. Clin Orthop Relat Res 1998;349:116–31.

23. Costigan W, Thordarson DB, Debnath UK. Operative management of ankle fractures in patients with diabetes mellitus. Foot Ankle Int 2007;28(1):32–7.

24. Schon L, Marks R. The management of neuroarthropathic fracture-dislocations in the diabetic patient - PubMed. Orthop Clin North Am 1995;26(2):375–92.

25. Dunn WR, Easley ME, Parks BG, et al. An augmented fixation method for distal fibular fractures in elderly patients: a biomechanical evaluation. Foot Ankle Int 2004;25(3):128–31.

26. Perry M, Taranow W, Manoli A, et al. Salvage of failed neuropathic ankle fractures: use of large-fragment fibular plating and multiple syndesmotic screws - PubMed. Surg Orthop Adv 2005;14(2):85–91.

27. Kaye RA. Stabilization of ankle syndesmosis injuries with a syndesmosis screw. Foot Ankle 1989;9(6):290–3.

28. Ayoub MA. Ankle fractures in diabetic neuropathic arthropathy. J Bone Joint Surg Br 2008;90(7):906–14.

29. Wallace SJ, Liskutin TE, Schiff AP, et al. Ankle fusion following failed initial treatment of complex ankle fractures in neuropathic diabetics. Foot Ankle Surg 2020; 26(2):189–92.

30. Johnson AR, Yoon P. Limb salvage in an unstable ankle fracture of a diabetic patient with Charcot arthropathy. Foot Ankle Spec 2010;3(4):184–9.

31. Ebaugh MP, Umbel B, Goss D, et al. Outcomes of primary tibiotalocalcaneal nailing for complicated diabetic ankle fractures. Foot Ankle Int 2019;40(12):1382–7.

32. Bazarov I, Peace RA, Lagaay PM, et al. Early protected weightbearing after ankle fractures in patients with diabetes mellitus. J Foot Ankle Surg 2017;56(1):30–3.

33. Rosenbaum AJ, Dellenbaugh SG, Dipreta JA, et al. The management of ankle fractures in diabetics: results of a survey of the American Orthopaedic Foot and Ankle Society membership. Foot Ankle Spec 2013;6(3):201–5.

34. Hedlund LJ, Maki DD, Griffiths HJ. Calcaneal fractures in diabetic patients. J Diabetes Complications 1998;12(2):81–7.

35. Kathol MH, El-Khoury GY, Moore TE, et al. Calcaneal insufficiency avulsion fractures in patients with diabetes mellitus. Radiology 1991;180(3):725–9.

36. Phyo N, Tang W, Kavarthapu V. Medium-term outcomes of multi-disciplinary surgical management of non-ischemic diabetic heel ulcers. J Clin Orthop Trauma 2021;17.

37. Athans W, Stephens H. Open calcaneal fractures in diabetic patients with neuropathy: a report of three cases and literature review. Foot Ankle Int 2008;29(10): 1049–53.

38. Sagray BA, Stapleton JJ, Zgonis T. Diabetic calcaneal fractures. Clin Podiatr Med Surg 2013;30(1):111–8.

39. Thorud JC, Plemmons B, Buckley CJ, et al. Mortality after nontraumatic major amputation among patients with diabetes and peripheral vascular disease: a systematic review. J Foot Ankle Surg 2016;55(3):591–9.

Limb Salvage in Severe Diabetic Foot Infection

Dane K. Wukich, MD*, Matthew J. Johnson, DPM, Katherine M. Raspovic, DPM

KEYWORDS

- Amputation • Diabetes • Foot • Infection • Limb • Preservation • Salvation

KEY POINTS

- Severe diabetic foot infections require admission to the hospital and prompt care.
- Acute surgical management of severe infection takes priority over advanced diagnostic workup.
- Major amputation is required in approximately 20% of patients and minor amputation in approximately 40% of patients.
- Because of underlying comorbidities, patients with severe diabetic foot infections are at risk for premature mortality.

INTRODUCTION

Severe diabetic foot infections (DFI) are both limb threatening and life threatening and associated with negative impact on health-related quality of life. Hospitalized patients with DFI self-reported significantly reduced mental and physical quality of life compared with patients with diabetes who did not have foot complaints.[1] Patients with diabetic foot disease such as Charcot neuroarthropathy, foot ulcers, and infections fear amputation more than death.[2] Consequently, DFI not only has a major impact on physical function but also creates increased emotional burden for patients and their families. The inpatient management of severe DFI is complex, and optimal care requires collaboration incorporating the skills of a multidisciplinary team.[3] In this Foot & Ankle Clinics issue, chapter 2 focuses on the importance and composition of a dedicated diabetic foot multidisciplinary team. Diabetic foot infections fall on a spectrum ranging from mildly infected foot ulcers to severe systemic infections, which can involve soft tissue only or have underlying osteomyelitis. Early diagnosis and treatment are paramount to preserve tissue, prevent limb loss, and maintain function. Initial treatment involves assessing the severity of infection, obtaining microbiological specimens, initiating appropriate antibiotic coverage, and determining if emergent surgical

University of Texas Southwestern Medical Center, 1801 Inwood Road, Dallas, TX 75390, USA
* Corresponding author. Department of Orthopaedic Surgery, University of Texas Southwestern Medical Center, 1801 Inwood Road, Dallas, TX 75391.
E-mail address: dane.wukich@utsouthwestern.edu

Foot Ankle Clin N Am 27 (2022) 655–670
https://doi.org/10.1016/j.fcl.2022.02.004
1083-7515/22/© 2022 Elsevier Inc. All rights reserved.

foot.theclinics.com

intervention is required. Severe DFIs require hospitalization, and in some cases, admission to critical care units due to metabolic and hemodynamic instability. Most severe DFIs require surgical intervention, and the goals of treatment should be preservation of limb function in addition to eradication of infection. Patients with DFI often have multiple comorbidities (cardiovascular, renal, neurologic, immunopathology) that increase the risk of morbidity and mortality. Using Kaplan-Meier methods, a single-center study reported that the cumulative mortality rates at 1 year, 5 years and 8 years of DFI patients were 5%, 22%, and 36%, respectively.[4] The Nuffield Trust recently reported the 5-year mortality rates of cancers in England, and the 5-year mortality rates in patients with DFI are worse than those in patients with testicular cancer, melanoma, prostate cancer, thyroid cancer, breast cancer, and Hodgkin lymphoma.[5] A holistic approach to treatment is necessary because the foot infection represents a surrogate marker of underlying illness in diabetic patients. For the purposes of this review, limb salvage is defined as avoiding amputation proximal to the transverse tarsal joint.[6] The definition of severe DFI is based on recommendations of the Infectious Disease Society of America (IDSA) and the International Working Group for the Diabetic Foot (IWGDF) and includes those patients who present with systemic inflammatory response syndrome.[7]

Outcomes of Severe Diabetic Foot Infection

A 2019 meta-analysis of DFI reported on risk factors for lower extremity amputation (minor and major). The investigators searched PubMed, Web of Science, and the Cochrane Trial Database and identified 6132 patients in 25 articles.[8] Nearly one-third of patients (1873 of 6132, 30.5%) underwent minor (at or distal to the transverse tarsal joint) or major lower extremity amputation (proximal to the transverse tarsal joint). Significant risk factors for lower extremity amputation included male gender, smoking, previous amputation, osteomyelitis, peripheral artery disease, retinopathy, severe infections, gangrene, neuroischemic diabetic foot infections, leukocytosis, positive wound cultures, and isolation of gram-negative bacteria. Although this study did not discriminate between moderate and severe infections, or minor and major amputations, it provides useful guidance for surgeons treating severe DFIs. During preparation of this manuscript, 5 studies over the past 10 years reported outcomes of severe DFI, including minor amputation, major amputation, and length of hospitalization.[6,9–12] Cumulatively, these 5 studies reported outcomes on 323 patients with severe DFI. Minor amputations were performed in 136 of 323 patients (42%), major amputations were performed in 70 of 323 patients (22%), and 206 of 323 patients (64%) required some form of amputation. The average length of hospitalization ranged from 8 to 19 days, although one study did not report length of stay.[12]

Diagnosis of Infection

Virtually all DFIs occur in patients with active wounds that begin with bacterial colonization. Lavery and colleagues[13] reported that 150 of 151 patients (99%) with DFI had a preexisting wound or penetrating trauma. Clinical signs of inflammation define the presence of infection in patients with foot wounds.[7] According to the IWGDF, at least 2 of the findings as listed in **Table 1** must be present: edema/induration, erythema, local tenderness or pain, warmth, or the presence of purulent drainage. Neuropathy, peripheral artery disease, or compromise of the immune system can moderate the clinical manifestations of inflammation in patients with diabetes. Significant risk factors for developing DFI include penetrating traumatic wounds, wound duration greater than 30 days, recurrent wounds, wounds that probed to bone, and presence of

Table 1 Diabetic foot infection classification system	
Clinical Classification of Infection	**IWGDF (IDSA) Classification**
Infection requires ≥ 2 or more of edema or induration • Periwound cellulitis • Tenderness or pain • Localized warmth • Purulent discharge	
Infection with no systemic manifestations (see later) involving (not any deeper tissues) and a periwound cellulitis < 2 cm	2 (mild infection)
Infection with no systemic manifestations and involving periwound cellulitis extending ≥2 cm and/or involving tissues deeper than skin and subcutaneous tissues (eg, tendon, muscle, joint, and bone)	3 (moderate infection)
Any foot infection with associated systemic manifestations (of the systemic inflammatory response syndrome [SIRS]), as manifested by ≥ 2 of the following: • Temperature, >38 C or <36C • Heart rate, >90 beats/min • Respiratory rate, >20 breaths/min or $Paco_2$ < 4.3 kPa (32 mm Hg) • White blood cell count >12,000/mm^3, or <4000/mm^3, or >10% immature (band) forms	4 (severe infection)
Infection involving bone (osteomyelitis)	Add "(O)" after 3 (moderate) or 4 (severe)

Adapted from the Infectious Disease Society of American and the International Working Group for the Diabetic Foot.

peripheral artery disease.[13] Wounds that probed to bone (odds ratio [OR] 6.7) and wounds older than 30 days (OR 4.7) were associated with the highest odds of DFI.

A thorough history and physical examination are critical for proper diagnosis, treatment, and achieving satisfactory outcomes. It is important to identify systemic signs of illness such as fever, chills, hypotension, tachycardia, unexplained hyperglycemia, nausea, vomiting, and anorexia.[7] The presence of these signs and symptoms, individually or collectively, raises the index of suspicion for severe infection. One of the earliest signs of infection in patients with active diabetic foot ulcers is unexplained hyperglycemia that differs from normal baseline. A 2013 study of hospitalized patients reported mean admission serum glucose of 300 mg/dL and 173 mg/dL in severe and moderate DFIs, respectively (P < 0.01). At the time of discharge the serum glucose was 150 mg/dL and 153 mg/dL in severe and moderate infections, respectively (P = 0.73).[6] The physical examination must document the perfusion status of the limb (presence or absence of pulses, gangrene) given the higher prevalence of peripheral artery disease in patients with diabetic foot disease.[14] Vascular studies (ankle-brachial index and toe pressures) and/or consultation with a specialist (vascular surgery, interventional radiology, or cardiology) experienced in lower extremity revascularization is appropriate in patients with an abnormal vascular examination or tissue loss associated with critical limb ischemia. The presence or absence of neuropathy (absent monofilament, absent vibration, or absent deep tendon reflexes) identifies patients at higher risk for infection. Severe nonpainful DFI indicates profound neuropathy and can delay presentation. Increase or development of pain in a patient with neuropathy and a diabetic foot wound should raise the index of suspicion for infection. Thoroughly inspect the wound and record length, width, and depth. The probe to bone test assesses wound depth and the likelihood underlying osteomyelitis.[15] Bullae, tissue necrosis, ecchymosis, petechiae, and/or crepitation are findings that herald the possibility of limb and life-threatening infections. Patients should have radiographs of both the foot and ankle to assess for foreign bodies, fractures, and the presence or absence of gas. Subcutaneous and/or deep fascial emphysema demonstrated on foot and ankle radiographs requires more proximal imaging of the leg. Waiting for advanced imaging (eg, MRI or noninvasive arterial testing) should not delay emergent surgical debridement, because time equals tissue. The acute surgical management of severe infection takes priority over advanced diagnostic workup.

Laboratory testing includes a complete blood count, comprehensive metabolic profile, and inflammatory markers such as erythrocyte sedimentation rate and C-reactive protein (CRP). Serum procalcitonin (PCT) is also biomarker of bacterial infection, and elevated PCT positively correlates with the severity of DFI[16] and independently predicts major amputation and in-hospital mortality.[17] A recent study identified several laboratory markers that were significantly different in patients with severe versus moderate infection. Serum albumin and hemoglobin levels were significantly lower in severe infections, whereas white blood cell count, erythrocyte sedimentation rate, CRP, and neutrophil/lymphocyte ratio were significantly higher.[10]

At presentation, obtain blood cultures and deep tissue specimens for microbiological analysis. Sterile collection of tissue using a curette or biopsy is preferred over superficial wound swabs. Broad-spectrum antibiotic coverage begins immediately in the emergency department after collection of microbiological specimens from both blood and wound. In the acutely infected setting, it is not necessary to delay antibiotics before obtaining definitive bone cultures in the operating theater. Withholding antibiotics before bone cultures has not demonstrated increased bacterial pathogen yield in DFI if osteomyelitis is present, and outcomes of patients with osteomyelitis are often worse.[18,19]

Severity of Infection

The IWGDF, incorporating recommendations from the Infectious Disease Society of America, has defined severity of infection.[7] Mild infections involve the skin and subcutaneous tissues with periwound erythema less than 2 cm, whereas moderate infections are associated with deeper infection (tendon, muscle, joint, bone, or fascia) and associated with periwound erythema greater than or equal to 2 cm. What distinguishes severe infection from moderate infection is the presence of systemic inflammatory response syndrome (SIRS) as illustrated in **Table 1. Fig. 1**A, B, and C illustrate clinical and radiographic findings of a patient who presented with leukocytosis, fever, and tachycardia. Edema, erythema, tissue necrosis, bullae formation (plantar and dorsal), and subcutaneous emphysema are consistent with a severe DFI, which is limb threatening.

The use of SIRS to distinguish moderate infections from severe infections was reported in hospitalized patients in 2013.[20] Patients with SIRS criteria had a 2.5 increased risk of any amputation (toe, foot, or above ankle) and a 7 times increased risk of major amputation compared with patients with moderate DFI. In addition, the length of hospitalization was nearly 4 days longer in patients with severe DFI. A more recent study from another institution reported that the need for surgery, amputation, duration of antibiotics, or healing rates within 1 year were not significantly

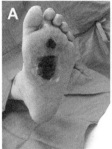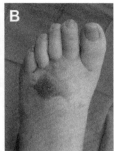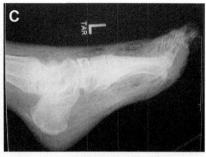

Fig. 1. (*A*) Plantar foot photograph of a patient who presented with leukocytosis, fever, and tachycardia. Note the presence of edema, erythema, and tissue necrosis and bullae formation. (*B*) Dorsal foot photograph of a patient who presented with leukocytosis, fever, and tachycardia. Note the presence of edema, erythema, and bullae formation. (*C*) Lateral foot radiograph of same patient as depicted in Fig. 1A and B subcutaneous emphysema, consistent with a severe DFI, which is limb threatening.

different between those with severe DFI (defined by SIRS) versus moderate DFI.[11] The length of hospital stay was significantly longer in patients with severe DFI (median 12.7 vs 7.8 days, P = .02) The major difference between the results of the 2 studies described is that the former study included patients with osteomyelitis (66%) and the latter study excluded those with osteomyelitis (0%).

An important contribution of the most recent IWGDF guidelines recognized that osteomyelitis might influence outcomes of DFI. Previous classifications did not discriminate whether or not osteomyelitis was present. If osteomyelitis is present, "O" is added to the classification such as IWGDF 4-O. For the purposes of this manuscript, the focus will be on severe DFI (IWGDF 4), in other words, those infections associated with SIRS. A recent study by Aragon-Sanchez and colleagues[21] reported that severe DFIs with osteomyelitis were not associated with worse outcomes (limb loss, loss of hospital stay, duration of antibiotic treatment, recurrence of the infection, and time to healing) compared with patients with only soft tissue DFIs. Nineteen percent of patients with severe infection underwent major amputation, and 36% of patients underwent minor amputation, with a combined amputation rate of 66%. Another study suggested reassessing the IDSA infection classification after discriminating between soft tissue infection and osteomyelitis.[22] There were no significant differences in moderate and severe soft tissue infection outcomes except for infection readmissions (46% vs 25%; P = .02) and acute kidney injury (31% vs 50%; P = .03). Similarly, the only significant differences in moderate and severe osteomyelitis admissions were the number of surgeries (2.8 vs 4.1; P < .01) and length of stay (19 vs 28 days; P < .01).

Surgeons should be familiar with other wound classifications that are relevant to patients with diabetic foot wounds. The Meggitt-Wagner Classification is the original wound classification and assesses depth, infection, and gangrene.[23] The University of Texas Classification (UT) assesses depth, infection as well as signs of ischemia. This matrix classification was superior to the Meggitt-Wagner Classification in predicting healing and risk of amputation.[23,24] SINBAD (site, ischemia, neuropathy, bacterial infection, and depth) creates a severity scoring scale.[24] Leese and colleagues[24] performed an observational study of greater than 1000 patients and found that SINBAD and University of Texas Classification were similar in predicting outcomes. PEDIS (perfusion, extent, depth, infection, and sensation)[25,26] and WIfI (wound, ischemia, foot infection)[27] are also commonly cited by scholarly work in this area. A prospective study compared the University of Texas, SINBAD, Meggitt-Wagner, and the PEDIS scoring systems. All classifications had satisfactory interrater agreement; however, the strength of the agreement varied between classifications. The Meggitt-Wagner system had an almost perfect agreement; the SINBAD and UT systems had a strong interrater agreement, and the PEDIS had a moderate interrater agreement.[28] The Society of Vascular Surgery developed WIfI to assist in the management of critical limb ischemia and created 3 mobile apps to facilitate use.[29]

Treatment

Empirical parenteral antibiotics should be started as soon as possible and include coverage for gram-negative and gram-positive organisms. Macerated wounds or wounds in patients from tropical climates may require coverage for Pseudomonas. Differences in climate, such as summer and winter, influence the type of bacteria that colonize diabetic foot ulcers.[30] The most commonly identified organisms in a meta-analysis of 112 studies of DFIs were *Staphylococcus aureus* (including methicillin-resistant *S aureus* [MRSA]), *Escherichia coli*, and Pseudomonas. Another interesting finding of this meta-analysis was that Gross National Income of countries significantly predicted the prevalence of gram-positive and gram-negative infections ($P < 0.0001$). Microbial isolates from high-income countries, classified by Gram staining, identified 62% gram-positive organisms and 38% gram-negative organisms, whereas isolates from low-income countries demonstrated 40% gram-positive organisms and 60% gram-negative organisms. Necrotizing fasciitis, ischemic infections, or gas-forming infections require anaerobic coverage as well. The need for MRSA coverage varies based on geography and local, institutional experience. Patient risk factors for MRSA include recent or prolonged hospitalization, recent nursing home stay, recent antibiotic use, hemodialysis, or long-term indwelling catheter or venous access. Antibiotic stewardship is important to mitigate growing antibiotic resistance.[31]

Initial Surgery

Thorough drainage of abscesses and debridement of necrotic tissue are the goals of the initial surgery. Knowledge of tissue planes and angiosomes assists in guiding incision placement, and all incisions should be extensile (**Fig. 2** reproduced with permission).[32] Three main source arteries supply 6 different angiosomes of the foot and ankle: the posterior tibial artery supplies the medial ankle and the plantar foot, the anterior tibial artery supplies the dorsum of the foot, and the peroneal artery supplies the anterolateral ankle and part of lateral hind foot (**Fig. 3** reproduced with permission).[33] The terminal branches of the posterior tibial artery each supply distinct portions of the plantar foot: the calcaneal branch supplies the medial heel, the medial half of the foot by the medial plantar artery, and the lateral half of the foot by the lateral plantar artery. The hallux is supplied by branches of both the medial and lateral plantar arteries as well as a branch of the dorsalis pedis. The terminal branches of the peroneal artery supply the anterolateral ankle (anterior perforating branch and lateral hindfoot [calcaneal branch]). The anterior tibial artery supplies the anterior ankle and then continues as dorsalis pedis artery. Choke vessels are important connections between 2 adjacent angiosomes and are critical to maintain perfusion if a source artery is damaged. Many patients with diabetic foot infections have peripheral artery disease and in some cases critical limb ischemia. In these patients collateral flow arising from an adjacent angiosomes may perfuse the ischemic part of the foot. The dorsal and plantar angiosomes of the foot communicate via an anastomosis between the dorsal pedis and lateral plantar artery through the proximal first interspace. Consequently, incision placement should minimize the risk of injuring a patent source artery

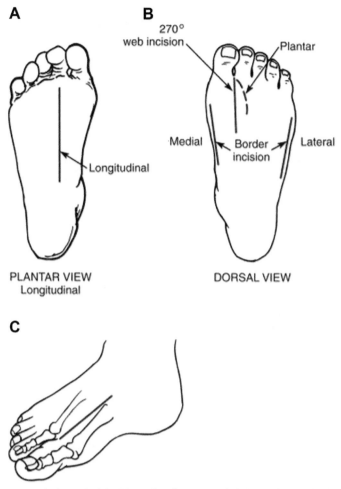

Fig. 2. Recommended surgical incisions for drainage of diabetic foot infections. (Reproduced with permission from Johnson JE, Klein SE, Brodsky JW. Diabetes. In: Coughlin MJ, Saltzman CL, Anderson RB, eds. Mann's Surgery of the Foot and Ankle. Vol 2 Figure 27-67, p 1444. Elsevier Saunders; 2014.[32])

and its choke vessels. Attinger and colleagues[34,35] provide an excellent review of angiosomes and their importance. Both references provide useful guidance on the principles of angiosomes to make safe incisions in patients with normal perfusion and those with vascular compromise. Infections tend to follow the path of least resistance, which is usually along tendons and tendon sheaths. Plantar medial infections can ascend into the medial or posterior leg following the long flexors of the hallux and lessor toes through the tarsal tunnel. Plantar lateral infections can ascend into the lateral and posterior leg compartments following the peroneal tendons. Dorsal infections ascend along the course of the long extensors of the toes and hallux as well as the tibialis anterior. The use of a tourniquet is at the discretion of the surgeon; however, inflation of the tourniquet may impede the ability to assess tissue viability. Limb elevation, as opposed to use of an Esmarch bandage, is preferred for exsanguination to avoid proximal spread of infection. If possible, design plantar foot incisions from an

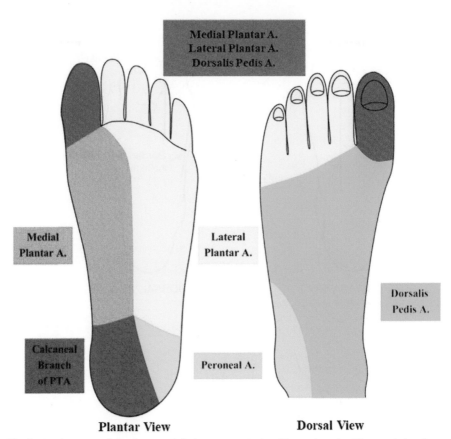

Plantar View   **Dorsal View**

Fig. 3. Angiosomes of the foot and their source arteries. (Reproduced with permission from Bekeny JC, Alfawaz A, Day J, et al. Indirect Endovascular Revascularization via Collaterals: A New Classification to Predict Wound Healing and Limb Salvage. Annals of vascular surgery. 2021;73:264-272.[33])

angiosomal perspective recognizing that both the medial plantar source artery and lateral plantar source artery are providing blow flow to each side of the incision. Thorough, but careful, debridement preserves viable soft tissue (skin or muscle) that facilitates definitive reconstruction and closure. Debridement should continue until normal tissue is encountered, demonstrated by healthy muscle that bleeds (red); healthy adipose tissue (yellow); and healthy tendons, fascia, or bone (white).[36] Plan incisions considering the future strategies for secondary closure or need for advanced reconstructive techniques. Exploration deep to the fascial layer is mandatory to identify a deep abscess. The compartmental anatomy of the foot is complex, and the exact number of compartments is a source of debate. More than 40 years ago, Loeffler and Ballard[37] identified 5 plantar fascial spaces. In 1990, Manoli and Weber[38] identified 9 compartments of the foot. As illustrated in **Fig. 4** (reproduced with permission),[39] these compartments include medial, superficial, lateral, forefoot (adductor and 4 interossei), and hindfoot. The medial, lateral, and superficial compartments run the entire length of the plantar foot, whereas the forefoot houses the adductor and 4 interossei compartments. The hindfoot compartment communicates with the deep posterior compartment of the leg, serving a portal of entry for foot infections to spread

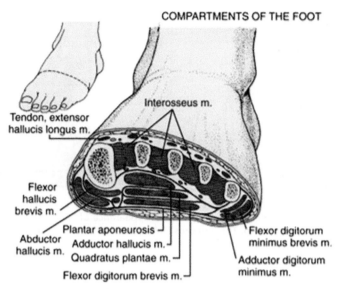

COMPARTMENTS OF THE FOOT

Tendon, extensor hallucis longus m.

Interosseus m.

Flexor hallucis brevis m.

Plantar aponeurosis

Abductor hallucis m.

Adductor hallucis m.

Quadratus plantae m.

Flexor digitorum brevis m.

Flexor digitorum minimus brevis m.

Adductor digitorum minimus m.

Fig. 4. Cross-sectional view of the compartments of the foot. (Mubarak SJ, Hargens AR. Compartment syndromes and Volkmann's contracture. Philadelphia: WB Saunders; 1981.)

proximally.[38] Any concern for proximal extension and ascending infection merits leg fasciotomies and exploration. Thorough wound irrigation further reduces bacterial load and removes cellular debris and exudate. The investigator prefers gravity irrigation with at least 3 L of normal saline using cystoscopy tubing. Povidone-iodine or prophylactic antibiotics can be added into the irrigation solution if the surgeon desires but has not shown decrease in bacterial yield in animal studies.[40] Wound management consists of packing the wound open or using negative pressure wound therapy. Loose approximation of surgical extensile incisions proximal and distal to the infected wound is reasonable in those patients with healthy tissue and a planned return to the operating theater. Significant bleeding can occur after debridement, and meticulous hemostasis is important. During subsequent surgery, methylene blue application to the wound is helpful to guide satisfactory debridement. The goal is to see only healthy tissue (red, yellow, and white) after the methylene blue dye is no longer visible[36] **(Fig. 5)**.

Local Antibiotic Delivery Systems

Despite thorough drainage and debridement, surgeons should presume that residual infection remains. After debridement of severe infections, particularly those complicated by bone resection, tissue loss may result in dead spaces. These cavities can be relatively hypoperfused, serving as an ideal site for hematoma and seroma formation. Systemic antibiotics may not deliver adequate concentrations of antibiotics in dead spaces. Local delivery systems result in high wound antibiotic concentration of antibiotics without systemic toxicity levels, which is relevant in patients with DFI because many have concomitant renal or hepatic impairment. Historically, the use of local antibiotic delivery systems arose from our colleagues in total joint arthroplasty and musculoskeletal infections. Polymethylmethacrylate (PMMA, bone cement) impregnated with antibiotics is an important tool in managing dead spaces associated with osteomyelitis. The limitations of PMMA as a carrier include a short period of

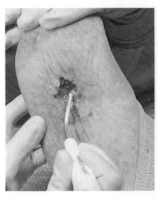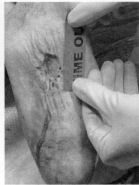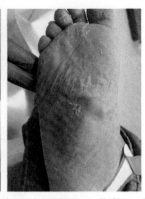

Fig. 5. Application of methylene blue dye to a wound before debridement (*left*) and appearance after debridement (*center*). The final appearance of the wound after healing is illustrated in the right photo. The 2 photos (*left* and *center*) were taken intraoperatively and the foot was painted with povidone-iodine solution. The photo on the right was taken in the outpatient clinic.

therapeutic antibiotic release (48–72 hours), need for removal, and potential for biofilm formation.[41] Autogenous bone grafting is not an ideal carrier in patients with DFI, and more recently synthetic bone graft substitutes, also known as biodegradable ceramic biocomposites have emerged. Resorbable bone substitutes mitigate the need for removal and include calcium sulfate, calcium phosphate (tricalcium phosphate), hydroxyapatite, and bioglass.[42]

Ideal local antibiotic delivery systems in patients with DFI are biocompatible, resorbable, and capable of delivering high therapeutic concentrations of antibiotics. In some cases, a carrier that provides mechanical bone support and the potential for osteoconduction is important as well. The rapid dissolution of calcium sulfate (6 weeks in soft tissue and 12 weeks in bone) results in high concentrations of local antibiotics during the immediate postoperative period. Because of the quick dissolution, calcium sulfate is not an optimal osteoconductive agent and has the potential for protracted sterile wound drainage. Calcium sulfate beads have advantages compared with PMMA, such as carrying a wider range of antibiotics, being completely biodegradable, and not requiring a second surgery for removal. A retrospective study of 137 cases of osteomyelitis (N = 127) or soft tissue infection (N = 10) was recently reported.[43] The protocol included surgical debridement and application of antibiotic impregnated calcium sulfate beads (Stimulan Rapid Cure, Biocomposites, Keele, Staffordshire, UK). Nearly 90% of infections resolved and 16% of patients did not require postoperative systemic antibiotics. Eighty percent of the wounds healed, with an average healing time of 11 weeks.

In an effort to decrease sterile drainage associated with calcium sulfate beads, combination bioceramics (also known as polyphasic synthetic bone substitutes) have gained popularity. These include combinations of β-tricalcium phosphate/calcium sulfate and hydroxyapatite/calcium sulfate bioceramics. An in vivo study demonstrated that the combination beads of β-tricalcium phosphate/calcium sulfate (Genex, Biocomposites Ltd., Keele, Staffordshire, UK) displayed similar efficacy compared with the calcium sulfate beads (Stimulan Rapid Cure, Biocomposites Ltd., Keele, Staffordshire, UK).[44] In addition to preventing and significantly reducing biofilm secondary to *Pseudomonas aeruginosa* and *S aureus*, β-tricalcium phosphate/calcium sulfate impregnated with antibiotics has potential to stimulate osteogenesis through acting as a scaffold.[44]

Calcium sulfate-hydroxyapatite bioceramics function as both a bone void filler and a local delivery system for antibiotics. A multicenter study using calcium sulfate-hydroxyapatite (Cerament G; BoneSupport, Lund, Sweden) reported wound healing in 84% of patients and treatment success in 66% (wound healing and no recurrence of osteomyelitis).[45] Another study of calcium sulfate hydroxyapatite (Cerament G; BoneSupport, Lund, Sweden) reported an overall healing rate of 81%; however, more proximal lesions had lower rates of success (~60% in the calcaneus and 70% in the tarsal bones).[42]

Bioactive glass is effective in treating osteomyelitis due to its antibacterial properties. Release of silicon, sodium, calcium, and phosphorus ions after implantation leads to local elevation of elevated pH and osmotic pressure.[46] In addition to antimicrobial properties, bioactive glass has angiogenic properties.[47] The calcium and phosphate molecules create a hydroxyapatite scaffold, allowing osteoblasts to migrate to the scaffold. Manipulation of the composition of bioactive glass can encourage bone formation and angiogenesis. A recent bioactive glass (S53P4 BonAlive Biomaterials, Biolinja 12 Turku, Finland) study of diabetic foot osteomyelitis reported significantly higher resolution rates and reduced need for antibiotics compared with conventional treatment.[48] Although not specifically targeting diabetic foot osteomyelitis, Romano and colleagues[49] reported that bioactive glass (S53P4 BonAlive Biomaterials, Biolinja 12 Turku, Finland) without local antibiotics demonstrated similar efficacy and less drainage than chronic osteomyelitis treated with 2 different antibiotic-loaded calcium-based bone substitutes.

Perioperative Care

Patients hospitalized with severe DFI require the expertise of a multidisciplinary, collaborative team for optimal medical and surgical outcomes. Internists or endocrinologists provide optimal management of perioperative hyperglycemia. Comorbidities of cardiac and renal disease often require consultation with cardiologists and nephrologists, respectively. Significant peripheral artery disease associated with critical limb ischemia requires intervention by vascular surgeons, interventional radiologists, or interventional cardiologists based on local availability of lower extremity intervention expertise. The precise duration, choice, and method of delivery (oral or parenteral) of antibiotics are beyond the scope of this surgical treatise, as is the definitive treatment of osteomyelitis beyond the acute setting. There is debate on the duration of antibiotic treatment, the route of antibiotic administration, and the need for "clean" surgical margins. One retrospective study in 2019 found no difference in recurrence of infection between patients with a "clean margin" versus those without, who underwent minor amputation for osteomyelitis.[50] Infectious disease consultation should guide the antibiotic regimen based on microbiological cultures.

Plastic surgeons offer skills that span the reconstructive ladder, ranging from skin grafting and local flaps to microsurgical free flap coverage. Before definitive reconstruction, whether using bioengineered tissue or autogenous tissue, the wound bed must be healthy, clean, and well perfused. The durability of split-thickness skin grafts on the plantar aspect in diabetic patients is not well studied. Recently, the Georgetown University Limb Salvage Team reported on 182 split-thickness skin grafts of the foot, most of which had diabetes (71%).[51] They found that plantar skin grafts (N = 52, 49 with diabetes) had significantly lower rates of healing at 60, 90 and 365 days compared with nonplantar skin grafts. Of those that healed, no significant difference in recurrence rates was observed at 1 year (plantar, 17% vs nonplantar 10%, $P = 0.17$). Reasons cited for avoiding plantar skin grafts are nondurability and breakdown; however, this study reported similar rates of breakdown compared with nonplantar grafts at 1 year. Many bioengineered tissues are accessible to wound care specialists, but autogenous skin grafting is widely available to surgeons and may be an option in carefully selected patients. Another report from the Georgetown University Limb Salvage Team reviewed their experience with microsurgical lower extremity free flap surgery in diabetic limb salvage surgery.[52] Immediate flap success was 94%, and long-term successful limb salvage was achieved in 78% of patients. Significant risk factors associated with failure include end-stage renal disease (OR 30.7), positive wound cultures (OR 6.1), hindfoot wounds (OR, 4.6), and elevated hemoglobin A1C level greater than 8.4% (1.4).

Wound care specialists, to include nurses and providers, are valuable consultants who assist in transition from the inpatient to outpatient setting. Dieticians and nutritionists are often helpful, as severe DFI is associated with protein depletion and negative nitrogen balance. The challenge is to restore nitrogen balance without inducing further hyperglycemia. Serum albumin is an acute phase reactant, and low serum levels indicate severe sepsis and inflammation.[6,10] Prealbumin levels are a better marker of nutrition during the immediate perioperative period. Finally, physical and occupational therapists are critical team members who facilitate restoration of function and activities of daily living.

Sequelae

Thorough debridement of necrotic soft tissue and bone often results in anatomic distortions, which can affect function of the foot and ankle; this occurs when certain tendons or their osseous insertions require excision to eradicate infection. For example, resection of the base of the fifth metatarsal or debridement of the peroneus brevis tendon contributes to varus deformity as a result of unopposed pull of the posterior tibial tendon. Sacrifice of the peroneus longus results in unopposed pull of the tibialis anterior, elevating the first ray creating forefoot varus. Both of these scenarios transfer load to the lateral column of the foot, predisposing to wound development. Sacrifice of the short and long toe flexors and extensors contribute to deformities of the hallux and lessor toes. Loss of the tibialis anterior function contributes to increased forefoot pressure secondary to unopposed gastrocsoleus contracture. Finally, loss of Achilles tendon function results in a calcaneus gait that predisposes the hindfoot to recalcitrant plantar ulceration. It is acknowledged that infection control is critical; however, when sacrificing important tendons in the foot and ankle, surgeons should consider the possibility of tendon balancing and realignment at some future state. Arthrodesis of the foot and/or ankle may ultimately be necessary to create a durable, stable, and plantigrade platform to maintain function.

SUMMARY

Severe DFIs are both limb threatening and life threatening and associated with negative impact on health-related quality of life. Patients with DFI often have multiple comorbidities (cardiovascular, renal, neurologic, immunopathology) that increase the risk of morbidity and mortality. Significant risk factors for lower extremity amputation include male gender, smoking, previous amputation, osteomyelitis, peripheral artery disease, retinopathy, severe infections, gangrene, neuroischemic DFIs, leukocytosis, positive wound cultures, and isolation of gram-negative bacteria. The acute surgical management of severe infection takes priority over advanced diagnostic workup. The presence of SIRS distinguishes severe infection from moderate infection. Bullae, tissue necrosis, ecchymosis, subcutaneous emphysema, petechiae, and/or crepitation are findings that herald the possibility of limb and life-threatening infections. Thorough drainage of abscesses and debridement of necrotic tissue are the goals of the initial surgery. Patients hospitalized with severe DFI require the expertise of a multidisciplinary, collaborative team for optimal medical and surgical outcomes. Once discharged from the inpatient setting, patients require vigilant follow-up. Postdischarge management may require advanced wound care, further surgical debridement, and future reconstructive surgery. Close inspection and surveillance of the contralateral "healthy" foot is necessary. The healthy foot experiences increased pressure and shear forces during the recovery process and is at risk for breakdown as well.

CLINICS CARE POINTS

- Microbiological specimens of the wound and blood guide antimicrobial therapy.
- Patients with severe DFI can present with severe metabolic and/or hemodynamic instability requiring intensive care admission.
- Management of acute infection takes priority over acute ischemia.
- Plan surgical incisions based on extensile incisions that incorporate knowledge of angiosomes and arterial anatomy.
- The acute hospitalization for DFI is only a part of the journey. Postdischarge follow-up may require advanced wound care, further surgical debridement, and future reconstructive surgery. Close inspection and surveillance of the contralateral "healthy" foot is necessary because it is at risk for skin ulceration and neuropathic arthropathy due to increased demands.

DISCLOSURE

D.K. Wukich is a consultant for Orthofix and Stryker Wright Medical, receives royalties from Arthrex, an Executive Board Member and President, International Association of Diabetic Foot Surgeons and a member of the Scientific Advisory Board for Advanced Oxygen Therapy, Inc. K.M. Raspovic is a consultant for Orthofix. M.J. Johnson has nothing to disclose.

REFERENCES

1. Raspovic KM, Wukich DK. Self-reported quality of life and diabetic foot infections. J Foot Ankle Surg 2014;53(6):716–9.
2. Wukich DK, Raspovic KM, Suder NC. Patients with diabetic foot disease fear major lower-extremity amputation more than death. Foot Ankle Spec 2018;11(1): 17–21.
3. Wukich DK, Armstrong DG, Attinger CE, et al. Inpatient management of diabetic foot disorders: a clinical guide. Diabetes Care 2013;36(9):2862–71.
4. Aragon-Sanchez J, Viquez-Molina G, Lopez-Valverde ME, et al. Long-term mortality of a cohort of patients undergoing surgical treatment for diabetic foot infections. an 8-year follow-up study. Int J Low Extrem Wounds 2021. 15347346211009425.
5. How does five-year cancer survival in England vary by cancer type? Nuffield-Trust. 2021. Available at: https://www.ons.gov.uk/peoplepopulationand community/healthandsocialcare/conditionsanddiseases/bulletins/cancers urvivalinengland/stageatdiagnosisandchildhoodpatientsfollowedupto2018. Accessed October 15, 2021.

6. Wukich DK, Hobizal KB, Brooks MM. Severity of diabetic foot infection and rate of limb salvage. Foot Ankle Int 2013;34(3):351–8.

7. Lipsky BA, Senneville E, Abbas ZG, et al. Guidelines on the diagnosis and treatment of foot infection in persons with diabetes (IWGDF 2019 update). Diabetes Metab Res Rev 2020;36(Suppl 1):e3280.

8. Sen P, Demirdal T, Emir B. Meta-analysis of risk factors for amputation in diabetic foot infections. Diabetes Metab Res Rev 2019;35(7):e3165.

9. Aragon-Sanchez J, Viquez-Molina G, Lopez-Valverde ME, et al. Surgical diabetic foot infections: is osteomyelitis associated with a worse prognosis? Int J Low Extrem Wounds 2021. 1534734620986695.

10. Aragon-Sanchez J, Viquez-Molina G, Lopez-Valverde ME, et al. Clinical, microbiological and inflammatory markers of severe diabetic foot infections. Diabet Med 2021;38(10):e14648.

11. Ryan EC, Crisologo PA, Oz OK, et al. Do SIRS criteria predict clinical outcomes in diabetic skin and soft tissue infections? J Foot Ankle Surg 2019;58(6):1055–7.

12. Kim BS, Choi WJ, Baek MK, et al. Limb salvage in severe diabetic foot infection. Foot Ankle Int 2011;32(1):31–7.

13. Lavery LA, Armstrong DG, Wunderlich RP, et al. Risk factors for foot infections in individuals with diabetes. Diabetes Care 2006;29(6):1288–93.

14. Wukich DK, Raspovic KM, Suder NC. Prevalence of peripheral arterial disease in patients with diabetic charcot neuroarthropathy. J foot Ankle Surg 2016;55(4):727–31.

15. Lam K, van Asten SA, Nguyen T, et al. Diagnostic accuracy of probe to bone to detect osteomyelitis in the diabetic foot: a systematic review. Clin Infect Dis 2016;63(7):944–8.

16. Zakariah NA, Bajuri MY, Hassan R, et al. Is procalcitonin more superior to hs-CRP in the diagnosis of infection in diabetic foot ulcer? Malays J Pathol 2020;42(1):77–84.

17. Meloni M, Izzo V, Giurato L, et al. Procalcitonin is a prognostic marker of hospital outcomes in patients with critical limb ischemia and diabetic foot infection. J Diabetes Res 2019;2019:4312737.

18. Crisologo PA, La Fontaine J, Wukich DK, et al. The effect of withholding antibiotics prior to bone biopsy in patients with suspected osteomyelitis: a meta-analysis of the literature. Wounds 2019;31(8):205–12.

19. Lavery LA, Ryan EC, Truong DH, et al. Does antibiotic treatment before bone biopsy affect the identification of bacterial pathogens from bone culture? Presentation 81st Scientific Sessions Am Diabetes Assoc Diabetes 2020;69.

20. Wukich DK, Hobizal KB, Raspovic KM, et al. SIRS is valid in discriminating between severe and moderate diabetic foot infections. Diabetes Care 2013;36(11):3706–11.

21. Aragon-Sanchez J, Lazaro-Martinez JL, Hernandez-Herrero C, et al. Surgical treatment of limb- and life-threatening infections in the feet of patients with diabetes and at least one palpable pedal pulse: successes and lessons learnt. Int J Low Extrem Wounds 2011;10(4):207–13.

22. Lavery LA, Ryan EC, Ahn J, et al. The infected diabetic foot: re-evaluating the infectious diseases society of america diabetic foot infection classification. Clin Infect Dis 2020;70(8):1573–9.

23. Oyibo SO, Jude EB, Tarawneh I, et al. A comparison of two diabetic foot ulcer classification systems: the Wagner and the University of Texas wound classification systems. Diabetes Care 2001;24(1):84–8.

24. Leese GP, Soto-Pedre E, Schofield C. Independent observational analysis of ul-cer outcomes for sinbad and university of texas ulcer scoring systems. Diabetes Care 2021;44(2):326–31.

25. Bravo-Molina A, Linares-Palomino JP, Vera-Arroyo B, et al. Inter-observer agree-ment of the Wagner, University of Texas and PEDIS classification systems for the diabetic foot syndrome. Foot Ankle Surg 2018;24(1):60–4.

26. Chuan F, Tang K, Jiang P, et al. Reliability and validity of the perfusion, extent, depth, infection and sensation (PEDIS) classification system and score in pa-tients with diabetic foot ulcer. PLoS One 2015;10(4):e0124739.

27. Vera-Cruz PN, Palmes PP, Tonogan L, et al. Comparison of WIFi, university of texas and wagner classification systems as major amputation predictors for admitted diabetic foot patients: a prospective cohort study. Malays Orthop J 2020;14(3):114–23.

28. Camilleri A, Gatt A, Formosa C. Inter-rater reliability of four validated diabetic foot ulcer classification systems. J Tissue Viability 2020;29(4):284–90.

29. Society of Vascular Surgery. Society for vascular surgery launches mobile apps for staging of chronic limb-threatening ischemia [press release]. Rosemont, Ill: Society of Vascular Surgery; 2020.

30. Dorr S, Freier F, Schlecht M, et al. Bacterial diversity and inflammatory response at first-time visit in younger and older individuals with diabetic foot infection (DFI). Acta Diabetol 2021;58(2):181–9.

31. Siddiqui AH, Koirala J. Methicillin resistant staphylococcus aureus. In: StatPearls. Treasure Island (FL): StatPearls Publishing; 2021.

32. Johnson JE, Klein SE Brodsky JW. Diabetes, In: Coughlin M.J., Saltzman C.L. and Anderson R.B., Mann's Surg Foot Ankle, vol. 2, 2014, Elsevier Saunders; Philadel-phia, PA, 1444, Figure 27-67.

33. Bekeny JC, Alfawaz A, Day J, et al. Indirect endovascular revascularization via collaterals: a new classification to predict wound healing and limb salvage. Ann Vasc Surg 2021;73:264–72.

34. Attinger CE, Evans KK, Bulan E, et al. Angiosomes of the foot and ankle and clin-ical implications for limb salvage: reconstruction, incisions, and revascularization. Plast Reconstr Surg 2006;117(7 Suppl):261S–93S.

35. Clemens MW, Attinger CE. Angiosomes and wound care in the diabetic foot. Foot Ankle Clin 2010;15(3):439–64.

36. Endara M, Attinger C. Using color to guide debridement. Adv Skin Wound Care 2012;25(12):549–55.

37. Loeffler RD Jr, Ballard A. Plantar fascial spaces of the foot and a proposed sur-gical approach. Foot Ankle 1980;1(1):11–4.

38. Manoli A 2nd, Weber TG. Fasciotomy of the foot: an anatomical study with special reference to release of the calcaneal compartment. Foot Ankle 1990;10(5):267–75.

39. Mubarak SJ, Hargens AR. Compartment syndromes and Volkmann's contracture. Philadelphia: WB Saunders; 1981.

40. Howell JM, Stair TO, Howell AW, et al. The effect of scrubbing and irrigation with normal saline, povidone iodine, and cefazolin on wound bacterial counts in a guinea pig model. Am J Emerg Med 1993;11(2):134–8.

41. Ferguson J, Diefenbeck M, McNally M. Ceramic biocomposites as biodegrad-able antibiotic carriers in the treatment of bone infections. J Bone Jt Infect 2017;2(1):38–51.

42. Whisstock C, Volpe A, Ninkovic S, et al. Multidisciplinary approach for the management and treatment of diabetic foot infections with a resorbable, gentamicin-loaded bone graft substitute. J Clin Med 2020;9(11).

43. Morley R, Rothwell M, Stephenson J, et al. Complex foot infection treated with surgical debridement and antibiotic loaded calcium sulfate-a retrospective cohort study of 137 cases. J Foot Ankle Surg 2021;61(2):239–47.

44. Jiang N, Dusane DH, Brooks JR, et al. Antibiotic loaded beta-tricalcium phosphate/calcium sulfate for antimicrobial potency, prevention and killing efficacy of Pseudomonas aeruginosa and Staphylococcus aureus biofilms. Sci Rep 2021;11(1):1446.

45. Hutting KH, Aan de Stegge WB, van Netten JJ, et al. Surgical treatment of diabetic foot ulcers complicated by osteomyelitis with gentamicin-loaded calcium sulphate-hydroxyapatite biocomposite. J Clin Med 2021;10(2).

46. Kojima KE, de Andrade ESFB, Leonhardt MC, et al. Bioactive glass S53P4 to fill-up large cavitary bone defect after acute and chronic osteomyelitis treated with antibiotic-loaded cement beads: A prospective case series with a minimum 2-year follow-up. Injury 2021;52(Suppl 3):S23–8.

47. Day RM. Bioactive glass stimulates the secretion of angiogenic growth factors and angiogenesis in vitro. Tissue Eng 2005;11(5–6):768–77.

48. De Giglio R, Di Vieste G, Mondello T, et al. Efficacy and safety of bioactive glass s53p4 as a treatment for diabetic foot osteomyelitis. J Foot Ankle Surg 2021; 60(2):292–6.

49. Romano CL, Logoluso N, Meani E, et al. A comparative study of the use of bioactive glass S53P4 and antibiotic-loaded calcium-based bone substitutes in the treatment of chronic osteomyelitis: a retrospective comparative study. Bone Joint J 2014;96-B(6):845–50.

50. Johnson MJ, Shumway N, Bivins M, et al. Outcomes of limb-sparing surgery for osteomyelitis in the diabetic foot: importance of the histopathologic margin. Open Forum Infect Dis 2019;6(10):ofz382.

51. Walters ET, Pandya M, Rajpal N, et al. Long term outcomes of split-thickness skin grafting to the plantar foot. J Foot Ankle Surg 2020;59(3):498–501.

52. Kotha VS, Fan KL, Schwitzer JA, et al. Amputation versus free flap: long-term outcomes of microsurgical limb salvage and risk factors for amputation in the diabetic population. Plast Reconstr Surg 2021;147(3):742–50.

Minor Forefoot Amputations in Patients with Diabetic Foot Ulcers

Oliver Michelsson, MD[a],*, Erkki Tukiainen, MD, PhD[b]

KEYWORDS

• Foot amputation • Toe amputation • Diabetes

KEY POINTS

- Limb-saving surgery.
- Good treatment of diabetes and vascularity.
- Timing of surgery.
- Amputation levels.
- Treatment after amputations.

Diabetic foot can lead to several pathophysiological changes, such as ischemia, neuropathy, deformities, or disturbed muscle balance and their combinations. These can start processes leading to forefoot amputations. Clinically, the changes observed in the distal foot present as loss of mobility, malposition of joints or bones, callosities, ulcers, distal gangrene, soft-tissue infection, and osteomyelitis.

The prevalence of diabetes mellitus, particularly type 2 diabetes, is increasing worldwide. The incidence of both lower limb revascularizations and amputations is increasing. However, more revascularizations are performed endovascularly, and the incidence of transtibial amputations is declining, whereas the incidence of toe and foot amputations is increasing.[1] This shift from transtibial amputations to partial foot amputations is regarded as an indicator of improved diabetes care and emphasizes the importance of foot amputations.

HISTORY

Limb amputations are among the oldest surgical procedures. In ancient times, they could be lifesaving procedures but possessed many complications and high mortality.

[a] Terveystalo Helsinki, Univeristy Hospital of Helsinki Porkkalankatu 22A, 00240 Helsinki, Finland; [b] Department of Plastic Surgery, Univeristy Hospital of Helsinki, Topeliuksenkatu 5, 00260 Helsinki, Finland
* Corresponding author.
E-mail address: oliver.michelsson@terveystalo.com

Foot Ankle Clin N Am 27 (2022) 671–685
https://doi.org/10.1016/j.fcl.2022.05.003
1083-7515/22/© 2022 Elsevier Inc. All rights reserved.

Artificial limbs, such as a forked stick, have been used since the beginning of mankind. As early as the first century, Celsus described an amputation.

A major step in the development of the operative technique was the introduction of artery forceps by Paré during the sixteenth century. Two famous amputation surgeons a pioneer of urology François Chopart (1743–1795) and gynecologist and also surgeon Jacques Lisfranc de St. Martin (1787–1847) have given their names to foot joint, Lisfranc and Chopart joints, and their own amputation lines for injured French soldiers in foot before anesthesia. Anesthesia was introduced in 1846 in Massachusetts general hospital USA, which contributed to the development of surgery allowing more complex and time-consuming procedures, and also lifesaving amputations. Russian surgeon Nikolay Ivanovic Pirogov (1810–1881) was the first to use anesthesia in field operations and developed different amputation techniques. The advance in medicine and surgical specialties and the introduction of the team approach improved the treatment and many patients can be treated without amputations.

CLINICAL EXAMINATION

Clinical examinations of the foot include always the inspection of the skin, also the interdigital areas, and posture of the foot during weightbearing. The warmth and color of the skin, pulses, sensation (10 g filament), and nail capillary reaction are checked. It is important to evaluate possible callosities and other signs of changes in skin suggesting overloading or early ischemic changes which may lead to diabetic ulcers or infection. The mobility of the joints, alignment of the foot in weight-bearing, and Achilles' tendon tightening (Silversköld test) are evaluated. Signs of critical ischemia are shiny, smooth, dry skin, thickening of toenails, no pulses, ulcers, infections, or dry gangrene (**Fig. 1**).

Native Xrays are always taken. They reveal the anatomy of the foot. However, osteomyelitis may become evident only after 2 to 4 weeks. For this reason, should be performed if any infection, osteomyelitis, or Charcot foot is suspected. C-reactive protein (CRP), red cell sedimentation rate, and leukocyte count are often helpful, but sometimes within the normal range in the early stage of a deep infection. Analysis of the HbA1c and glucose is used to evaluate long-term glucose control to optimize the treatment of diabetes for better wound healing.

Ankle-brachial pressure index (ABI) can be used in diabetic patients, but the values should be interpreted with caution. Sensitivity of the standard threshold of 0.9, which is conventionally used to define peripheral vascular disease, seems to be lower in diabetic patients with complications. Also, the frequent arterial wall calcifications present in diabetes tend to increase ABI. It has been shown that ABI values of more than 1.3 are correlated with peripheral arterial disease. Therefore, ABI less than 0.9 and more than 1.3 are highly suspicious for arterial disease in patients with diabetes.[2] Toe pressure measurement is a good adjunct to evaluate the distal arterial perfusion. Intraarterial digital subtraction angiography (DSA) is the gold standard for lower limb arterial imaging. It is an invasive procedure but allows the possibility to perform endovascular revascularization. It may also guide the level of amputation and help in the planning the skin flaps according to the vitality of tissues on each side of the foot.

ACUTE DIABETIC FOOT INFECTION

An acute diabetic foot infection can be a serious condition. It is the leading cause of hospitalization and amputation in patients with diabetes. The onset of infection can be insidious due to neuropathy. In acute infection, early surgery is often mandatory as soon as the diagnosis is evident and the general condition of the patient is adequate. Acute invading infection demands rapid antibiotic treatment at the same

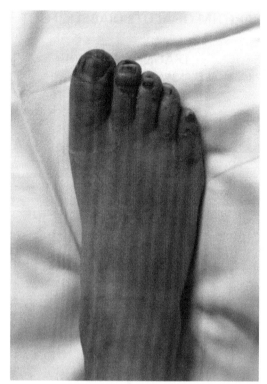

Fig. 1. Acute diabetic infection and typical findings in acute ischemia. Shiny, smooth, dry skin of the foot, thickening of the toenails, open sores, skin infections, ulcers, and dry gangrene (*black toes*).

time the patient is being prepared for surgery by treating disturbed glucose metabolism, dehydration, and decreased renal function. Once the general condition allows, new wound excisions, decompression, or amputation is performed.

TIMING

Chronic ulcers and dry gangrenes usually do not need acute surgery. The patient is evaluated (medical evaluation, angiography, MRI, the need for revascularization) and the treatment of diabetes is optimized. In differential diagnosis, Charcot foot can be challenging to differentiate from infection. **Fig. 2** Logarithm.

Soft-tissue Surgery

Wound excision (debridement) of the foot lesions should follow the basic surgical rules. These include the relief of excessive tension in tissues, drainage of collections, and removal of dead and severely infected tissues.

The excision of skin should be limited to the minimum and vital "unanatomical" skin flaps or extensions should first be preserved. Slaps can be guided with angiography which shows the actual condition of foot arteries. This is important if transmetatarsal amputation is performed and the bone coverage or plantar surface needs durable cover.

If muscle is not bleeding, contracting or is discolored, it should be removed. Muscle compartments should be opened if the pressure is increased. Often infections spread

LOGARITHM OF ACUTE DIABETIC FOOT

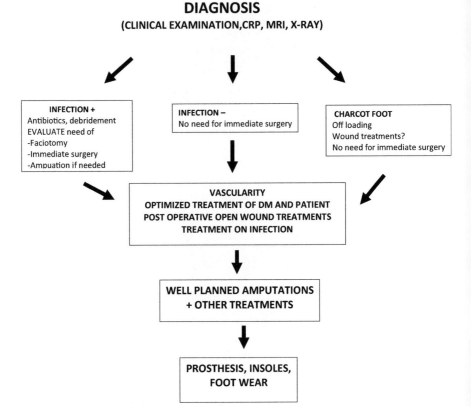

DIAGNOSIS
(CLINICAL EXAMINATION,CRP, MRI, X-RAY)

INFECTION +
Antibiotics, debridement
EVALUATE need of
-Faciotomy
-Immediate surgery
-Ampuation if needed

INFECTION –
No need for immediate surgery

CHARCOT FOOT
Off loading
Wound treatments?
No need for immediate surgery

VASCULARITY
OPTIMIZED TREATMENT OF DM AND PATIENT
POST OPERATIVE OPEN WOUND TREATMENTS
TREATMENT ON INFECTION

WELL PLANNED AMPUTATIONS
+ OTHER TREATMENTS

PROSTHESIS, INSOLES,
FOOT WEAR

Fig. 2. Logarithm of treating an acute diabetic foot in emergency care, timing treatments, and planning the amputation.

more proximally in the tendon sheaths. This may demand decompression or excision more proximally. Affected bones (long bones) should be resected using saw (not bone cutting instruments) to avoid crushing and further fractures of the distal bone ends.

In case of chronic diabetic wounds, the aim of debridement is to transform the biology of a chronic wound into that of an acute wound. Well performed debridement gives a chance of healing provided the oxygen demand of the tissue is met, the infection has been eliminated, and the patient is not catabolic. In most cases, it is safest to close or reconstruct the wound in a second operation (secondarily), when the general and local signs of infection and edema have subsided.

Negative pressure wound therapy (NPWT) is commonly applied as an adjunct in diabetic foot ulcers and it has several obvious advantages. It is used to prepare the fresh wound for closure and cover.[3] It protects the wound from nosocomial infections, diminishes tissue edema, promotes the granulation of the wound and prepares the wound for closure, and makes the wound care easier. However, it should not be used in inadequately excised infected wounds and it should not replace adequate surgical debridement. The quality of the tissue after prolonged NPWT is not stable enough, especially on the weight-bearing surface and such a wound can sustain wound breakdown. It may also disturb the circulation if applied circularly over a dysvascular distal foot.

Options for wound coverage/reconstruction are direct closure with skin flaps created during the amputation procedure, skin grafting and local, pedicular, or free flaps. Vital plantar skin is the best cover for the amputation stump, and it should be preserved when amputation is first performed. Skin grafts can be placed only on exposed vital fat, muscle, or granulation tissue. Skin grafts are not successful in covering exposed tendons or bones. Skin grafts are not durable on a plantar stump or on any the point of the foot that is exposed to continuous high pressure.

To cover the stump end or on the dorsal aspect of the foot local plastic surgical flaps often offer a solution. However, in distal, ischemic foot local or pedicled flaps raised just proximally of the amputation level are usually inadequate for wound coverage as there is only little viable tissue available due to infection, fibrosis, and most importantly their viability is very limited. Furthermore, failure can lead to the more extensive tissue defects.

Free tissue transfer can offer a solution in selected cases (**Fig. 3**). The circulation should be optimized by using an endovascular procedure or arterial bypass reconstruction.[4] In our experience, defects on the amputation end and dorsal foot can be covered with this method with good results. The free muscle flap or fasciocutaneous flap is microsurgical anastomosed either to a patent native artery on the foot/ankle or directly end-to-side to the bypass graft. If the distal anastomosis of the arterial bypass

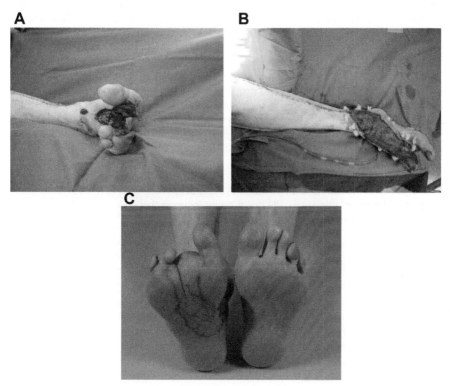

Fig. 3. (A): Picture after revision of the gangrene and bony resection of 2nd and 3rd rays. There is a large tissue defect. (B). Picture from surgery after the bypass surgery and the latissimus dorsi flap that will be covered with skin. (C). Late final postoperative results show the shrinkages of the flap and a useful extremity.

is not possible to a native artery in the foot/ankle, the free flap can be connected end-to-end to the bypass which gets into inflow popliteal and femoral artery (see **Fig. 2**). New vessels will grow between the free flap and the foot during the following weeks. This enhances the circulation in the foot.

DISTAL AMPUTATION LEVELS OF THE FOOT

This article covers the only forefoot and midfoot amputations. The minor foot amputation of foot include toe, ray, transmetatarsal, tarsometatarsal (Lisfranc), and transtarsal amputations (Chopart). Amputations need to be extensive enough to solve the underlying pathology. Amputation must be planned carefully thinking about the function of the foot and the possible problems which can ensue. The aim is to mainten the adequate bone length, proper contouring of bony elements. The skin and wound closure should be performed without tension using well perfused, proportionate, and durable soft tissue.

The main goal of forefoot is to maintain the ability to walk. Patients needs to get a plantigrade foot and a normal parabola of the forefoot to gain as normal function as we can in the.

An evaluation of the amputation is conducted carefully, we recommend a multiprotection approach, cooperation with a plastic surgeon (soft tissues), and orthopedic surgeon (function of the foot) and if needed, by a vascular surgeon and a diabetes specialist. Many hospitals in Finland have multidisciplinary meetings to evaluate and plan the treatments and timing for each diabetic patient. The amputation level should be extensive enough to allow soft-tissue healing and closure either directly or with reconstruction. The anticipated future function and presumed activity level of the limb do affect the level of amputations.

A plethora of tests have been suggested in the surgical and orthopedic literature as the "best" method to determine the proper level of amputation.[5] These procedures include arterial Doppler pressure measurements, fluorescein angiography, transcutaneous oxygen tension measurements, and xenon clearance.[5]

TOE AMPUTATIONS

Toes can be partially or totally amputated. The first ray and toe are important for the biomechanics of the foot and amputation of the first toe may lead to a mild dysfunction in the gait. However, this is usually not a major issue in this group of patients, especially if part of the proximal phalanx is saved (**Fig. 4**).

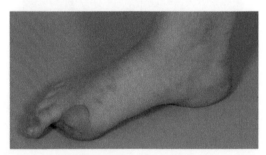

Fig. 4. Final postoperative result after partial I toe amputation. Insertion of I toe tendons, proximal part of phalanx is saved, and a fillet flap (skin flap from the toe) has been used for soft-tissue coverage. Notice the skin lesions of the second toe that needs to be addressed before a chronic ulcer or infection develops.

First toe exarticulation at the MTP-joint level can increase pressure at the remaining distal metatarsal bone leading to ulceration and infection, if not prevented with spacers. For this reason, many authors support preserving the basis of the first phalanx with the muscle insertions, if possible, to prevent this. The same kind of phenomenon is also possible after the removal of the whole fifth toe; the distal end of the fifth metatarsal, the bone end may become prominent and exposed. In those cases, partial distal resection of the MT has been suggested.

Single amputation of the third, fourth, or fifth toes is usually well-tolerated. However, a single toe amputation (2–4 toes) creates an empty space, and the adjoining toes tend to turn toward this leading to malposition. The removal of the second toe can lead to hallux valgus, if not prevented with a spacer. After the removal of 2 adjacent toes, the risk of malposition of the remaining toes is even greater. In general, if 2 to 4 toes are removed, leaving only 1 to 2 toes in place, we suggest transmetatarsal amputation. Single-standing toes are constantly exposed to minor trauma and later deformity, so they should be amputated **(Fig. 5)**. The big toe is an exception, because it is more valuable for the biomechanical function of the foot.

Sometimes even a partial toe amputation like Syme opertationn, ampuation of half or 2/3 of the distal phalanx with the nail, can be performed for a single toe distal gangrene.

RAY AMPUTATIONS

Single ray amputations are usually well-tolerated **(Fig. 6)**. After a single mid-ray amputation, the foot maintains usually its function in gait, its tripod (quadroid). Many surgeons leave the proximal part of the metatarsal intact.

Even 2 lateral rays can be removed, but this demands careful judgment and good patient compliance. This kind of foot requires usually an individual custom-made prosthesis.

Removal of 2 or more medial rays gives a poor result, both functionally and cosmetically.[6] In these cases, a more proximal amputation should be considered.

Lateral 2 rays (fourth and fifth) can be removed preserving a someway useful function. The same does not apply to the removal of the first ray, more than one ray in the middle (including the second, third, and fourth) should be performed only in exceptional cases. In these cases, a transtarsal or other proximal amputation is preferred directly. Amputations of the last (lateral) 2 rays increase the risk of developing adduct, varus, and supinated foot.[6] The distribution of the load is more balanced, because of the preservation

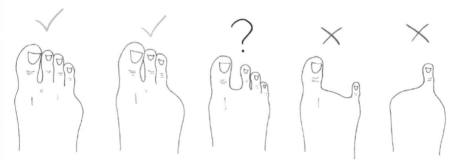

Fig. 5. You may amputate partially toes or single toes, or a group of toes. But never leave a single toe standing alone. Single toes are highly exposed to trauma and often develop malposition.

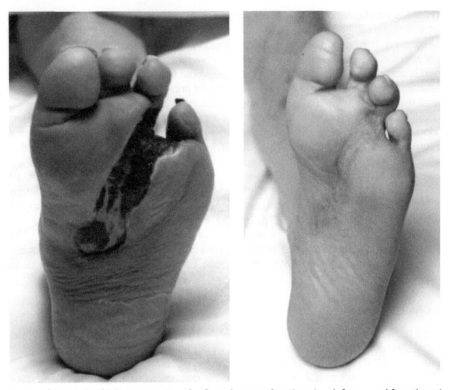

Fig. 6. After one mid-ray amputation the foot does not lose its tripod, form, and function. A Picture during the healing process after fourth ray amputation and B final result after healing.

of the first, second, and third ray, increasing the possibility of using orthoses, reducing the risk of ulceration, and a subsequent more proximal amputation.[6]

Any resection of metatarsal head can lead to transversal overloading of the unamputated bones to the adjoining MTP joint areas. This may cause new ulcers and soft-tissue problems. In first ray amputations, it is always preferable to leave the shaft as long as possible to aid the elevation of the medial arch and that way support with custom-molded inserts.[6] If any amputation, for example, extensive first ray amputation, extends proximal of the insertion of tibialis anterior, and the insertion needs to be reinserted to maintain the dorsiflexion.

It is important to remember is that during an amputation, especially when metatarsal bones involved, all plantar bone edges should be rounded. Fifth ray the shaft should be transected obliquely, and preserving the proximal part of the bone with insertion of the peroneus brevis. In the literature, you may find successful results after amputations of both the first and fifth ray (**Fig. 7**).

Transmetatarsal Amputation

Transmetatarsal amputation is to be performed if needed due to the level of gangrene, infection, or when more than 2 rays need to be amputated (**Fig. 8**). Transversal dorsal and plantar incision are made forming 2 flaps preserving the plantar skin as much as possible (**Fig. 9**). Bone is transected proximally from the incision allowing vital flaps to

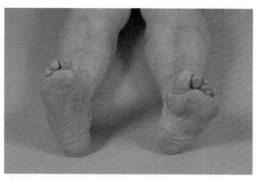

Fig. 7. Patient had both 1st and 5th ray amputated. This is the end results and patients are able to walk normally.

be closed without any tension. Optimally larger plantar flap should always cover the anterior parts and all of the weight-bearing area.

Optimally, the plantar durable skin flap (thick skin) should cover the weight-bearing areas totally. To provide maximum surface area on the foot for secure suspension of a shoe, it is important to save as much metatarsal shaft length as possible and covered it with good plantar skin for flap reconstruction.

If the amputation extends to the basis of all the 5 metatarsals, tendon attachments of the tibialis anterior and peroneus brevis on the first and fifth metatarsals should be preserved if possible, to maintain tendon balance, in both directions. Especially the function of tibialis anterior muscle, which antagonizes the triceps surae and Achilles's tendon, is essential to avoid the development of an unusable equinus foot. Tibialis anterior is also the primary inverter of the foot and peroneal tendons are evertors. Both these functions are needed to maintain muscle balance, inversion versus eversion.

We recommend that the amputation should follow the normal parabola of foot third, fourth, and fifth ray should be shorter than the first and the second [the Baroucks principles of forefoot] (**Fig. 10**). Also, the bone cuts should be performed using a saw, avoiding so that it will sharp plantar, lateral, or medial edges or any metatarsal protruding. Any bony prominence creates a high risk of ulcer which may lead to infections and more proximal amputations.

Removed metatarsal heads cause loss of load-bearing capacity, stability, and dynamic function. So, in younger and still active sporting patients in these cases a

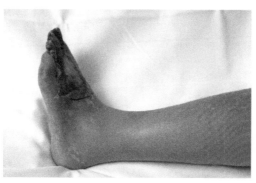

Fig. 8. Gangrene and infection have extended all the way to the metatarsal area of the foot and this patient needs TMA level amputation.

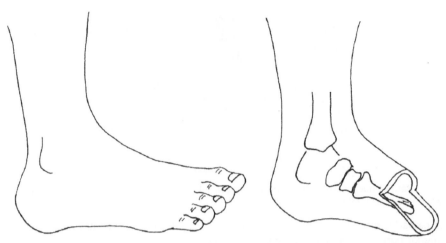

Fig. 9. Incision in transmetatarsal amputation. Large plantar flat should cover the loading area and bone edges.

more proximal, transtibial amputations are to be considered. However, in diabetes, there is a significant risk for a more proximal amputation or contralateral amputation. Age and diabetic neuropathy affect balance. Distal amputations of foot are always preferred to be more proximal in older less active diabetic patients than have a risk of contralateral amputations.

In TMA, to help maintain a balanced residual foot, the insertions of the peroneus brevis, peroneus longus, and anterior tibial tendons are preserved.

TARSOMETATARSAL (LISFRANC) AND CHOPART DISARTICULATION

Lisfranc joint was described by Lisfranc 1815. A Lisfranc disarticulation should be considered when the soft-tissue coverage of exposed bones is not possible or the previous amputation has failed (**Fig. 11**). TMA is preferred, nonfunctional partial fore-foot amputation, due that the better load-bearing capacity and stability.

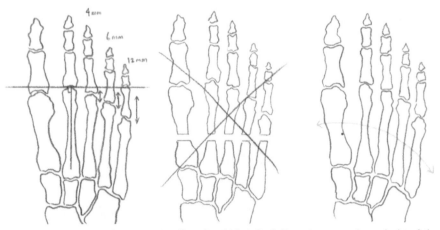

Fig. 10. Transmetatarsal amputation line should briefly follow the normal parabola of the foot, especially avoiding any protruding bone or bony edges.

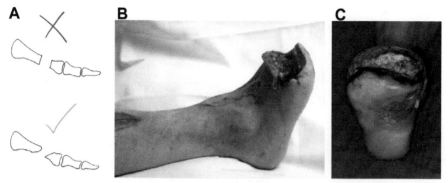

Fig. 11. (*A*) Never leave any sharp bony edges.(*B*) Well healing open wound. Red healthy good tissue and ready for final wound closure. (*C*) Poorly healing necrotic tissue and wound necrosis. Needs a more proximal amputation.

Lisfranc and Chopart amputations lead to reduced dynamic function and barefoot walking is impaired. However, when the infection extends proximally, disarticulation at the tarsometatarsal joint (Lisfranc joint,) or midtarsal (Chopart) is necessary. Again, good soft-tissue coverage of the load-bearing areas with the plantar flap is essential, like in TMA. Lisfranc amputation may require tendon balancing. To help maintain a balanced residual foot, the insertions of the peroneus brevis, peroneus longus, and anterior tibial tendons are preserved or transferred. Tibialis anterior insertion should always be reinserted in the middle of talus, and even other extensors like extensor hallucis longus or extensor digitorum longus can be used to reinforce extension. Tendon balance is always important, but especially if there already is existing joint stiffness or joint contracture.

If the residual foot is fed predominantly by an anterior tibial or peroneal artery, the Lisfranc amputation usually preserves the communication with the plantar arterial system through the first perforating branch. This arterial communication is destroyed in Chopart Amputations.

To help maintain a balanced residual foot, the insertions of the peroneus brevis, peroneus longus, and anterior tibial tendons are preserved or transferred.

ADDITIONAL PROCEDURES

Plantigrade foot, muscle, and tendon balance are essential for adequate function of the foot.

For diabetes, typically, an Achilles contracture develops, especially during long hospitalization. Achilles' contracture is to some extent possible to prevent with a simple splint or exercises.

Achilles tendon lengthening is required if foot is in the plantigrade position for protection of the distal foot area from extra pressure during gait. Proximal gastrocnemius fascia incision should be liberally performed. In the techniques described by Strayer or Bauman procedure, the incision placed is proximally, at the junction of upper and middle thirds of the lower leg, to avoid skin complications. In cases with more severe Achilles' tightening, percutaneous Achilles' elongation is to be preferred, it may cause some Achilles weakening.

Changes in the biomechanics and gait may require tendon transfers to address the possible development of forefoot varus. Typically, split tibialis anterior tendon transfer laterally or a peroneus brevis tendon transfer may be used.[7] Roukis and colleagues[8]

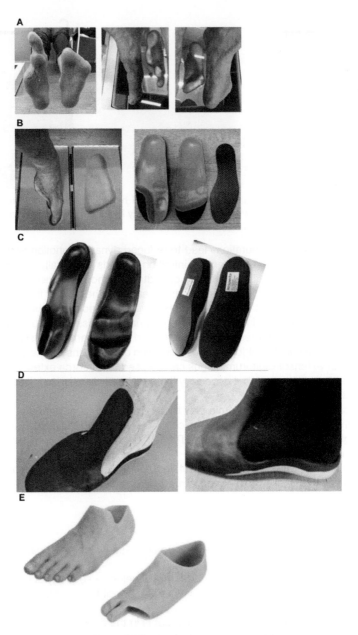

Fig. 12. With different insoles or parietal prosthesis, it is possible to get cosmetically and functionally a better foot. Insoles/prosthesis will improve the stability of the foot and enlarge the supporting area. (*A*) A patient with partly amputated feet. Right foot only 1st ray left, left foot all toes amputated from MTP level. Picture is from the first 3D planning session of the custom-made insoles. (*B*) Premanufactured models of the insoles. (*C*) Final insoles for both feet. (*D*) Example of special insoles with ankle supporting dorsal flap. (*E*). Silicone partial foot prosthesis is both functional but also esthetically looks like a normal foot.

Box 1
Indications Prosthesis for partly amputated parts of the foot

Amputation levels:
 Chopart
 Lisfranc
 Syme's amputation
 Transmetatarsal amputation
 Amputation of one or more rays of the foot
 Amputation of the big toe or several toes

---

described a flexor hallucis longus and extensor digitorum longus tendon transfer for balancing the foot following a TMA.

FOOTWEAR AND PROSTHESIS

After amputations, the optimal pressure distribution and gait should be supported with orthoses, modified footwear or so-called rocker bottom shoes. Surgeons should have a basic knowledge of how to support the foot with prosthesis after amputations (**Fig. 12**).

Foot prosthesis and footwear have 3 functions. The prosthesis should esthetically look like a foot. Secondly, mechanical factors improve the stability of the foot by creating a more rigid platform under the foot. It may enlarge the supporting area and play the part of the 3 points of the foot (and in some studies even 4 points, S. Meyes, 2019 quadpod).[9] Foot has such a great impact on balance so orthoses increase the supporting area of the foot and that way also may help to retain better overall balance. However, they will not replace the lack of proprioception due to the amputation of the foot parts and/or ankle. Contraindications for prosthesis are poorly healed stumps or open wounds. See **Box 1** for indications of insoles and prosthesis.

GAIT AFTER AMPUTATIONS

There are 8 phases of human gait and any change in the foot function or structure changes somehow the activities in these eight phases (**Box 2**). In the terminal stance, the heel is off the ground. It means that the whole bodyweight is supported by the forefoot and more accurately on the medial side of the forefoot. The stability of the medial

---

Box 2
Eight phases of human gait

1. Initial contact

2. Loading response

3. Midstance; early and late

4. Terminal stance

5. Preswing

6. Initial swing

7. Midswing

8. Terminal swing

---

arch is partly dependent on the windlass effect of the dorsiflexion of the toes. This combination is really hard to achieve with a prosthesis on an amputated foot.

In the preswing phase, the foot is reaching the point which is often referred to as forefoot rocker. In all 3 swing phases, the major purpose of any prosthesis or improvement of the footwear must ensure that the ground clearance is safe and the point of the shoe/foot is not hitting the ground and causing the person to stumble.

With the preservation of full leg length and a stable heel pad, the Chopart patient can walk with direct end bearing for short distances without a prosthesis. This short residuum has no direct rollover function. A custom-made rigid-ankle prosthesis or orthosis and a shoe with a rigid rocker bottom should be provided. If "drop foot" is secondary to nerve trauma, transfer of a posterior muscle-tendon unit may be added for its tenodesis effect, with an ankle-foot orthosis (AFO) fitted after wound healing.

SUMMARY

Minor forefoot amputations are becoming more common. Severe acute foot infection may indicate immediate surgery, but in other cases, careful patient evaluation, right timing for both the pre and postoperative treatments are essential to ensure adequate healing. It is important to anticipate the healing process and function when the level of amputation is decided. General risk factors are age, kidney function, circulation of the foot, and possible infection or Charcot deformity. The patients role is also essential; he should be well informed to be able to take part in the decision making. Amputations, even minor ones, are always irreversible and important for the patient. Amputations should be performed on the suitable level and if needed, using flaps for soft-tissue coverage (see **Fig. 2**). The aim is to get a well-balanced plantigrade foot with durable tissues.

CLINICS CARE POINTS

- Infection and ischemia in the diabetic foot are considered the 2 most significant threats to limb salvage.
- Lower limb amputation is a severe complication that causes physical impairment and affects negatively life expectancy.
- The level of amputation is a crucial choice influencing the physical and mental health status of the patient.
- Interest in limb salvage has grown during the last decades.
- The initiation of multidisciplinary groups and increased revascularizations and soft-tissue reconstructions cause a decrease in major amputations and an increase in limb salvage and distal amputations.
- More than 90% of patients who underwent multiple limb salvage attempts but eventually ended up having a major amputation, would still choose to undergo the attempts to save the leg (C.C. Hong, Tan JH, Lim SH, Nather A. Multiple limb salvage attempts for diabetic foot infections: is it worth it? Bone Joint J. 2017, 99 B(11):1502 to 1507.)
- Insufficient or delayed debridement can cause the infection to spread and cause extensive necrosis and increase the likelihood of amputation (Faglia E, Clerice G, Gaminiti M, Quarantiello A, Gino M, Morabite A. The role of early surgical debridement and revascularization in patients with diabetes and deep foot space abscess: Retrospective review of 106 patients with diabetes. J Foot Ankle Surg, 2006, 45, 220–226).

DISCLOSURE

The authors have nothing to disclose.

REFERENCES

1. Hughes W, Goodall R, Salciccioli JD, et al. Trends in lower extremity amputation incidence in European Union 15+ countries. 1990-2017. Eur J Vasc Endovasc Surg 2020;60(4):602–12.
2. Potier L, Abi Khalil C, Mohammedi K, et al. Use and utility of ankle brachial index in patient with diabetes. Eur J Vasc Endovasc Surg 2011;41(1):110–6.
3. Vikatmaa P, Juutilainen V, Kuukasjärvi P, et al. Negative pressure wound therapy: a systematic review of effectiveness and safety. Eur J Vasc Endovasc Surg 2008;36: 4238–48.
4. Tukiainen E, Kallio M, Lepäntalo M. Advanced leg salvage of the critically ischae-mic leg with major tissue loss by vascular and plastic surgeon teamwork: long-term outcome. Ann Surg 2006;244:949–58.
5. Kirker S, Ritchie J Chapter 5 - Amputations, Prostheses, and Rehabilitation of the Foot and Ankle. Core Top Foot Ankle Surg 2018.
6. Bowker John H. MD Partial Foot Amputations and Disarticulations: Surgical As-pects. JPO J Prosthetics Orthotics 2007;19(8):P62–76.
7. Schweinberger MH, Roukis TS. Soft-tissue and osseous techniques to balance forefoot and midfoot amputations. Clinpodiatr Med Surg 2008;25:623–639viii-ix.
8. Roukis TS. Flexor hallucislongus and extensor digitorumlongus tendon transfers for balancing the foot following transmetatarsal amputation. J Foot Ankle Surg 2009;48:398–401.
9. Winter DA. Foot trajectory in human gait. Phys Ther 1992;72(1):45–53.

Mid- and Hindfoot Amputations in Diabetic Patients

Martin C. Berli, MD, PD[a,b,*]

KEYWORDS

- Midfoot amputation • Hindfoot amputation • Lisfranc amputation
- Bona-Jaeger amputation • Chopart amputation • Spitzy-Pirogoff amputation
- Boyd amputation • Syme amputation

KEY POINTS

- Mid- and hindfoot amputations maintain the mobility of the patient on short distances without auxiliary means.
- The self-perception (body image) of the patient remains intact, which increases the acceptance of the surgical intervention.
- In mid-foot amputation no leg length discrepancy needs to be compensated, and in hindfoot amputations it depends on the type of surgery.
- Not all hindfoot amputations are appropriate for diabetic patients due to polyneuropathy and peripheral arterial disease.
- Getting on an adapted shoe or an ankle-foot orthosis is usually much easier for patients than getting on a prosthesis.

INTRODUCTION

Despite great progress in the treatment of diabetes mellitus, amputations are still a serious concern in the affected patients. This is mainly due to the diabetic comorbidities in long-term diabetic patients. The central complications are polyneuropathy (PNP) and peripheral arterial disease (PAD). Furthermore, the weakened immune system increases the risk of infection, which is due to a reduced intensity of the immune reaction.[1] The skin of these patients is altered mainly due to the reduced elasticity caused by a change in the collagen synthesis,[2] and the autonomous neuropathy, which reduces the sweat secretion leading to a dry skin and a tendency to develop

[a] Division of Technical Orthopaedics, Department of Orthopaedic Surgery, Balgrist University Hospital, Zurich, Switzerland; [b] Universitätsklinik Balgrist, Forchstrasse 340, 8008 Zurich, Switzerland
* Corresponding author. Universitätsklinik Balgrist, Forchstrasse 340, 8008 Zurich, Switzerland.
E-mail address: martin.berli@balgrist.ch

Foot Ankle Clin N Am 27 (2022) 687–700
https://doi.org/10.1016/j.fcl.2022.05.004
foot.theclinics.com
1083-7515/22/© 2022 Elsevier Inc. All rights reserved.

rhagades. They represent a breach in the physical defense barrier and increase the risk of infection, as they serve as an entrance for bacteria and fungi.[1,3]

Depending on the involved germs, and particularly on the time span until an ulcer or infection is detected, these patients need to undergo surgery. A well-known threat are major amputations, in particular the below-the-knee amputation (BKA).[4-7] The BKA represents a major handicap and results in approximately 20% of the patients with long-term diabetes in wheelchair dependency.[8]

If an infection is detected early, several techniques of mid- and hindfoot amputations are possible to maintain a maximum amount of the natural body.[9] Besides the maintained body image, minor amputations also allow energetically a better function, as the energy consumption increases significantly with every amputated joint.[10-13]The peripheral arteries in patients with long-term diabetes are often altered, and also the central arteries, leading to a diminished cardiac function and reduced general resilience.[14]

After the surgery, the patients need to be equipped with a prosthetic device. In the midfoot amputations, a void-filler in the front part of the shoe is often sufficient if it is produced with a laminated, rigid sole to avoid pressure of the device against the foot stump during the toe-off phase while walking.

The shorter the foot stump gets, the higher the prosthetic device needs to be. However, the Bellmann prosthesis is considered sufficient for amputations up to the Chopart joint.[10,15] For more proximal amputations of the lower extremity, a frame orthosis is needed with a strut on the proximal tibia to achieve a better distribution of the pressure and a more secure gait. In addition, in the more proximal amputations, the resulting leg length discrepancy needs to be compensated for long-distance walking, whereas short distances can be overcome without any auxiliary means.

MIDFOOT AMPUTATIONS

The following mid-foot amputations are commonly used surgical options and will be discussed in detail: Lisfranc-, Bona-Jaeger-, and Chopart-Amputation.[16-19]

Lisfranc Amputation

The Lisfranc amputation is named after a French gynecologist and military surgeon: Jacques Lisfranc (1790–1847).[20,21] Lisfranc described his "new surgical method for the partial amputation in the tarsometatarsal joint" as a surgical improvement opposed to the Chopart amputation, which was previously developed as a first step to preserve as much "healthy soft tissue as possible." Before Chopart, it was common to perform exclusively BKAs. Lisfranc being a military surgeon made his observations in the war between 1813 and 1814 and developed his new surgical method based on his findings. He made cadaveric studies and described meticulously a surgical method, which he considered safe against failing. His essay was received positively by the board of surgeons on May 1, 1815 in Paris and accepted as a new surgical method for partial foot amputations. The main indication for a Lisfranc amputation is extensive soft tissue loss, which prevents a successful transmetatarsal amputation.

It is performed along the so-called Lisfranc joint line, which runs along the tarsometatarsal joints (ossa cuneiformia, os cuboideum, and metatarsal bones) and marks the border between the mid-foot and the forefoot[22] (**Fig. 1**). In this type of amputation, the entire mid- and hindfoot remains intact, including the plantar skin, which results in an end-bearable stump with a maintained leg length. The surface of the stand is significantly higher than with the Chopart amputation, which increases the stability of the patient and eases the adaptation of the shoes. In these cases, an orthotic forefoot

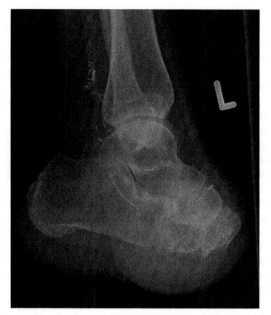

Fig. 1. Lateral radiography of a 29-year-old diabetic patient after a Lisfranc amputation.

replacement is usually sufficient, or as described by Roach and colleagues[22] a blocked-in forepart in normal footwear, without a stabilizing brace reaching above the ankle (**Fig. 2**). The investigators described in their study titled "Resurrection of the Amputations of Lisfranc and Chopart for Diabetic Gangrene" 18 successful amputations with either of these techniques in more than 6 years. His reasoning is similar to the one Lisfranc made in the early 1800s: the need for alternatives to BKA, which was the standard of care in the United States if an amputation was needed on the lower leg or the foot, but seemed exaggerated in certain cases, where only parts of the foot were concerned. Early writes in his article "Transmetatarsal and Middfoot Amputations": "Amputations at the Lisfranc and Chopart's joint levels have proven more difficult and until recently were out of favor. Initial problems with these midfoot amputation levels were the result of difficult shoe fit and positional malalignment of the residual limb, resulting in high complication rates and poor patient satisfaction. Recent advances in surgical technique and prosthetic fit have addressed these earlier problems."[23]

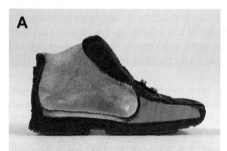
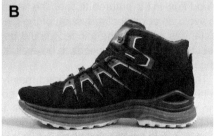

Fig. 2. Prosthetic device for a Lisfranc amputee.

With a careful surgical preparation, the insertions of dorsal extending foot muscles, the anterior tibial muscle, and the proximal insertion of the long peroneus muscle, both on the medial cuneiform, can be spared. With that, a malposition of the foot in an equinus position is less probable. A physical test of the dorsiflexion during surgery helps to estimate the balance of the remaining foot. In case of a limited dorsiflexion, a percutaneous lengthening of the Achilles tendon is a valuable treatment option.[5,24] Roach and colleagues[22] described in their small series that an equinus malposition did not occur, nor was a lengthening of the Achilles tendon necessary.

The tibialis posterior tendon inserts on the medial aspect of the navicular tubercle and extends to the plantar surface of all midfoot bones and the bases of the second and the third metatarsals.[23] This muscle provides inversion and plantar flexion power to the foot. It is only at the level of the metatarsal bases, Lisfranc joint, that various muscle attachments begin to affect the foot position.

There is a higher risk for a malposition of the foot stump in supination, in case the fifth metatarsal bone is completely removed and the pronating peroneus brevis tendon not transosseously fixed to the cuboid or the lateral cuneiform bone. For this reason, the base of the fifth metatarsal should be preserved, if possible.[25,26] Alternatively, Greene and Bibbo described a technique, where the insertion of the tibialis anterior tendon is preserved and the extensor hallucis tendon is transferred to the lateral cuneiform bone, which led to a more plantigrade stump and balanced range of motion. However, a consequent tendon balancing is definitely necessary for the biomechanical balance and the successful outcome of the midfoot amputations.

There is no unanimity concerning the removal of the cartilage surface of the joints. Bowker recommends the removal, particularly in infected situations, as cartilage is bradytrophic tissue and can serve as a nutrient medium for bacteria. On the other hand, by removing the cartilage coverage of the spongious bones, the intra- and postoperative bleeding is higher and the wound healing takes longer with a higher risk for a delayed wound healing. Another factor is the scarring: with the cartilage coverage of the tarsal bones, the soft tissue scar remains more mobile and flexible and therefore, the risk of ulcers or delayed wound healing is low. With the removed cartilage coverage of the tarsal bones, the soft tissue scar gets attached to the bones and loses its elasticity. With a rather fixed scar, the risk of ulcers increases.

The vascular situation in the Lisfranc amputation is particular, as for a stable and resistant soft tissue coverage of the joint line, a longer plantar flap out of plantar skin is formed and sutured to the dorsal skin of the foot, which is more fragile being of the field skin type. Owing to this coverage design, the plantar flap is bent dorsally. In case of calcified plantar arteries, their diameter diminishes, which reduces the blood flow to the periphery. Therefore, skin necrosis along the wound is typical in vascular patients. This needs to be considered during the suturing. Each stich diminishes the blood flow in the sutured tissue. The wound closure must be possible without tension to avoid an additional reduction of the diameter of the arteries in the plantar flap. The distances between the stiches should be as large as possible, and the necessity of subcutaneous sutures needs to be evaluated, all with the goal to minimize the interference with the blood flow.

The prosthetic device is needed mainly to replace the missing forefoot of the patient.[10,15] This is basically a void-filler combined with a rigid insole. Depending on the remaining length of the stump, the tendency to a supinated position, and the remaining mobility in the hindfoot, a more stable prosthetic device may be needed or the prosthesis needs to be combined with an orthopedic shoe with an ankle exceeding shaft.

Useful Modifications of the "Classic" Lisfranc Amputation

Bowker[5] considers the base of the second metatarsal bone as the "keystone" of the foot. Leaving its base in a Lisfranc amputation in place can help to preserve the proximal transverse arch.

The consequent amputation along the Lisfranc joint line can also lead to long-term wound healing problems because of the open joints with persistent synovia production as mentioned by Sanders and Early.[23,27] This complication can often be avoided by performing a transmetatarsal amputation slightly distal to the joint line.[27]

Bona-Jaeger Amputation

The surgical line in this type of amputation starts between the navicular and the cuneiform bones and extends straight through the cuboid bone by prolonging the line of the disarticulation. The surgery should be performed very carefully due to the anatomic position of the plantar arteries below the median and lateral cuneiform bones. In this type of surgery, the possible strength of the dorsiflexion is significantly diminished, in particular in comparison to the Lisfranc amputation. Therefore, a combined percutaneous lengthening of the Achilles tendon is often indicated to avoid an equinus malposition of the foot. Baumgartner describes as an alternative the possibility of a surgical fusion of the Chopart joints,[16] but only in patients without neural or vascular dysfunction, which is usually not the case in a population with diabetes (**Fig. 3**A–C).

The prosthetic device for the shoe remains the same like for transmetatarsal or Lisfranc amputations. Although the Bona-Jaeger procedure is generally known and accepted, there is no scientific literature supporting it.

Chopart Amputation

The Chopart amputation is named after François Chopart (1743–1795), a French urologist and surgeon in Paris. The procedure was first described in 1792 by Lafiteau.[20] At that time, Chopart's amputation technique was revolutionary, as all patients who needed to undergo surgery at the distal lower extremity including the foot were operated with a BKA. Chopart felt irritated by the fact, that in many cases of a BKA a major amount of healthy tissue was unnecessarily cut.

According to Roach approximately 50% of the patients with diabetes, who had to undergo amputational surgery, had another amputation on the opposite leg within 5 years.[22] Approximately one-third of the amputated patients were in that period unable or unwilling to wear or use a prosthesis. Therefore, the Chopart procedure was considered a helpful surgical technique to keep the patients mobile, for short distances even without a prosthetic device, as the leg length and the hindfoot are kept and a limited mobility of the ankle and the subtalar joints is maintained. Owing to a relatively high

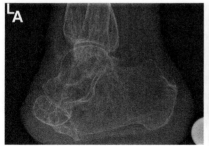
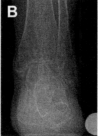
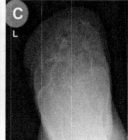

Fig. 3. (A) Lateral, (B) ap radiographs of the ankle joint, and (C) oblique radiography of a 59-year-old diabetic patient after a Bona–Jaeger amputation.

rate of complications and failures, this surgical technique was abandoned for quite some time, but was reactivated in the 1970s and 1980s with modified techniques.[22] Nowadays, it is part of the commonly recognized surgical techniques, although it is performed mostly in specialized centers.

The surgical technique presents as follows: the amputation line leads through the talonavicular and calcaneocuboid joints. The central step of the procedure is the section of the bifurcal ligament, which forms a functional unit between the calcaneus, the navicular and the cuboid bones. It is therefore considered the key ligament.

The main problem of the Chopart amputation is due to the fact that the dorsiflexors of the foot are completely removed, which leads to an increasing equine position of the remaining foot stump,[28,29] as there is no physical opposition to the triceps surae muscle. The increasing equinus position of the foot stump can be partially corrected with a lengthening of the Achilles tendon and a transosseous fixation of the anterior tibial tendon in the talus[5,24] that can even allow a little dorsiflexion of the remaining foot stump. Bowker describes the removal of 2 to 3cm of the Achilles tendon to be more effective, than simple lengthening. Leaving the sheath of the tendon in place allows a rapid reconstitution of its new length. To keep the new length of the tendon and prevent an equinus malposition of the stump, a total contact cast is applied for 6 weeks. This allows at the same time the healing of the transosseously fixed anterior tibial muscle. In an infected wound, the reinsertion of the poorly vascularized anterior tibial tendon with sutures, anchors or interference screws can, however, lead to new infected tissue and recurrent wound breakdown.

In this equine position, the anterior plantar process of the calcaneus becomes prominent and bears most of the weight, when the patient stands upright. This bony prominence is not covered by the heel fat pad, which moves proximally in the described position. A high risk of ulceration and infection is the resulting consequence, in particular in patients with neural or vascular dysfunction. This is the reason, why the mentioned bony prominence needs to be removed during surgery. For these reasons, the Chopart amputation is rarely performed in the diabetic patient[30–32] (**Fig. 4**A, B).

The skin flaps for the soft tissue coverage of the talus and the calcaneus are designed symmetrically. Bowker considers the removal of the cartilage of the joint surface necessary in case of an infection with the idea to lower the risk for bacterial survival in this bradytrophic tissue.

Concerning the vascular situation, the posterior tibial artery is central for a good outcome of the Chopart amputation.[33] The risk of necrosis in the heel pad increases significantly, if the posterior tibial artery is obstructed, as it is often the case in a vascular patient, the collateral vessels are insufficient for the supply of the entire stump. The dorsal artery of the foot is usually not strong enough to maintain the supply of the entire foot in case of an amputation.

The aforementioned postoperative treatment with a removable total contact cast (rTCC) keeping the foot in a plantigrade position followed by a custom-made off-loading ankle-foot orthosis (AFO) with a well-adapted footbed can help to reduce the risk of ulceration and failure of the treatment by avoiding an equinus position of the stump (**Fig. 5**). The crucial part of the AFO is the rigid plantar reinforcement. Biomechanically, this helps to increase the surface of the stand and prevents the dorsiflexion of the orthosis, which would lead to pressure ulcerations in the distal part of the stump.

A detail that is usually underestimated but crucial concerning the prevention of new skin ulcers: the socks. If the patient wears on both feet the same size of socks, he will sooner or later get blisters or ulcers due to the friction, as the excess of the sock will be squeezed between the stump and the prosthesis. The same problem is caused by seams. This is the reason why special Chopart-socks without seams are produced and should be prescribed by the responsible surgeon.

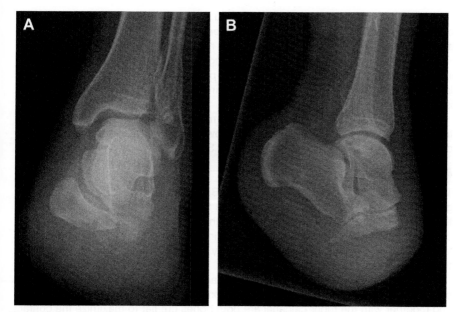

Fig. 4. (*A*) Ap and (*B*) lateral radiographs of a 62-year-old diabetic patient after a Chopart amputation.

HINDFOOT AMPUTATIONS

The following hindfoot amputations are rarely used in the diabetic patient since the remaining stump has a relatively small surface to distribute the pressure and is therefore prone to ulcerations, particularly in patients with a reduced sensitivity and vascular perfusion. A good perfusion of the posterior tibial artery is crucial for a good outcome in hindfoot amputations.

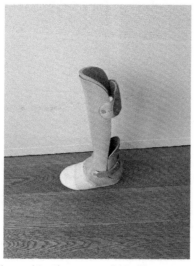

Fig. 5. AFO as it is typically used in Chopart- and hindfoot amputations.

Most of the specialized surgeons involved in the treatment of the diabetic foot consider hindfoot amputation in long-term diabetic patients with the typical comorbidities too risky and still perform in these cases rather a BKA.[34]

Another disadvantage is the resulting leg length discrepancy, which can lead to gait instability, falls, and chronic lumbar pain, if the patient walks too often without an auxiliary mean. Still, it is possible to walk short distances without a prosthetic device, which is a clear advantage over the BKA.

However, even if only performed in a limited number of situations, it is still necessary to know these options and therefore the following hindfoot amputations will be discussed in detail: Boyd-, Spitzy-Pirogoff-, and Syme-Amputation.[16,35]

Boyd Amputation

The Boyd amputation is named after Harold B. Boyd (1904–1981), an American surgeon . The goal of this surgical procedure is to create a weight-bearing surface of the heel by building an arthrodesis between the tibia and the calcaneus.[36] This procedure leads to the biggest surface of all hindfoot amputations. The resulting leg length discrepancy is usually at approximately 2–4 cm (**Fig. 6**A, B). The sensitivity of the heel and the heel pad are preserved.

Technically, this intervention consists in an exarticulation along the calcaneocuboidal joint and the removal of the talus. Next, the distal joint of the tibia is removed and together with the tuber calcanei are both bones cut flat to maximize the contact between them. There are different possibilities to achieve the aimed arthrodesis: the two bones can be fixed with an external fixator or with Kirschner wires or screws, or simply with an rTCC. The important point is to get a stable contact with a maximum pressure between the two bones, which allows them to unify.

The quality of the bone can be a problem until the amputation is performed. The patients are often immobile for a long period of time. The reasons are numerous, either because the patient has recurrent ulcerations, which need to heal with an off-loading

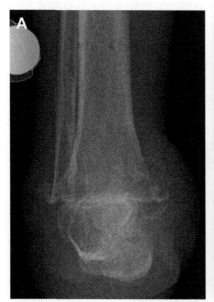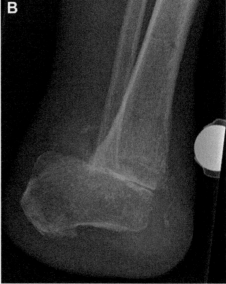

Fig. 6. (A, B) Ap and lateral radiographs of a 77-year-old diabetic patient after a Boyd amputation.

treatment, or because of the general health condition. Both reasons lead to an inactivity osteoporosis, which is a disadvantageous condition for an arthrodesis. External problems are possible, if the patient is a long-time smoker, if an infection is present or if the patients have long-term corticoid medication.

Another problem in these patients is the compliance[10]: as the patient needs to off-load the arthrodesis until it reached weight-bearing stability, a relatively high level of compliance is mandatory. This is particularly true in patients with the above-mentioned reduced quality of the bone stock, where the process of the bone healing needs significantly more time. Off-loading is also a problem in elderly patients, which are in a physically bad shape or simply deconditioned due to their general health situation.

The vascular situation is similar to the Chopart-amputation: the main artery for the perfusion of the concerned area is the posterior tibial artery. If its perfusion is limited for any reason, the wound healing after the operation is prolonged, which is not only true for the soft tissue but also for the arthrodesis. This is also true for potential new ulcers and needs to be monitored on a regular basis, for example, in the regular clinics.

Once the stump is healed and can be charged again, the patients need a custom-made AFO with a high shaft, a so-called ortho-prosthesis, especially designed for this kind of amputation. The important points are a compensation of the leg length discrepancy, a rigid inlay for the shoe with enough volume compensation to avoid a dorsiflexion of the shoe during gait. The AFO can be worn in a regular shoe and should correlate in size and volume with the opposite side.[11]

Spitzy-Pirogoff Amputation

The Pirogoff hindfoot amputation (1854) was initially developed by Nikolai Pirogoff (1810–1881), a Russian surgeon, with the idea to provide full-weight-bearing stumps and therefore allow a short ambulation without prosthesis.[37] The heel pad and the sensibility of the sole of the heel are preserved and a tibio-calcaneal arthrodesis is established (**Fig. 7**A, B). There are several modifications described to the original technique,

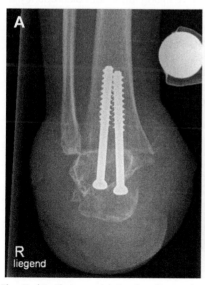
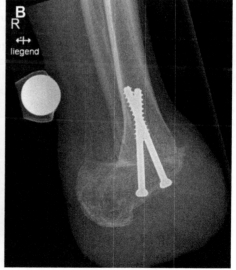

Fig. 7. (A, B) Ap and lateral radiographs of a 48-year-old diabetic patient after a Spitzy-Pirogoff amputation.

including Boyd—as described above—and others.[38] These modifications served to reduce the complication rates and improved the outcome.

Performing this procedure, the surgeon removes two-thirds of the calcaneus and leaves a relatively small part of the calcaneus to be fixed under the tibia.[38,39] The distal tibial joint surface is removed in order to create a surface, where a spongy bone contact is possible and a stable arthrodesis can be established.

The modification of this procedure by Hans Spitzy (Austria, 1872–1956) consists in leaving a bigger part of the calcaneus, which is rotated under the tibia after the talus is removed. The anterior part of the calcaneus is cut transversely in a 45° angle. Afterwards, the tibio-calcaneal arthrodesis is achieved by a stable fixation with either an internal fixation with screws or with an external fixator or a combination of both. The success of the procedure depends on the quality of the bone and the compliance of the patient. Big advantages of this procedure are the preservation of the heel fat pad and its sensitivity, and the minimal leg length discrepancy.[40]

However, Baumgartner does not recommend this kind of surgery in diabetic patients due to the high failure rate caused by a prolonged bone union time.[16]

The prosthetic device should be produced in form of an AFO, a higher shaft helps to increase the stability of the prosthesis and to distribute the pressure in order to avoid plantar ulceration. Ideally, the AFO should contain a well-adapted footbed to prevent local pressure peaks and support the cushioning effect of the heel pad (**Fig. 5**).

Syme Amputation

James Syme (UK, 1799–1870) described the radical amputation of the hindfoot with the removal of the talus, the calcaneus, and both malleoli[41,42] (**Fig. 8**A, B). The heel fat pad is moved under the resulting weight-bearing surface. Even if completely insensate, it is surprisingly activity tolerant, provided, that it is held firmly in place under the tibia. Precise prosthetic fitting is an absolute prerequisite.[4]

Owing to the relatively small footprint, there is a high risk of ulceration in neuropathic patients.[43]

The main disadvantage of this procedure is the resulting leg-length discrepancy of 4–7 cm, which needs to be compensated. Still, for short distances the patients are able to ambulate without auxiliary means, but only with severe limping. In order to be able to walk without fall, the equilibrium of these patient needs to be intact.

This kind of surgery is contraindicated in patients without a sufficient function of the posterior tibial artery, as the wound will not heal, and later on the risk for skin necrosis is severely elevated.[4] Owing to the reduced elasticity and sensitivity, there should be no scar in the heel pad, as the risk for ulceration would be significantly increased.

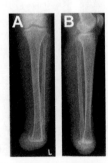

Fig. 8. (*A, B*) Ap and lateral radiographs of a 31-year-old diabetic patient after a Syme amputation.

These patients need an AFO with a long shaft, propping against the tibial tuberosity, including a compensation for the leg length discrepancy. As mentioned above, a tight-fitting prosthetic shaft keeping the heel pad consequently in place under the tibia is an absolute prerequisite to ensure a good long-term outcome.

GENERAL PECULIARITIES IN THE SURGERY OF THE DIABETIC FOOT

- Transosseous tenodeses can often not be performed due to the bad quality of the bone and ongoing soft tissue infection. Therefore, surgical procedures should be executed without this technique[44].
- Owing to the impaired vascular situation, surgical bone and soft tissue interventions should be performed with minimal damage, as the healing capacity of these patients is very limited. This diminishes the possibility of surgical corrections and adaptations during the main procedures.[45]
- The surgery in diabetic patients should be planned in a way that the soft tissue coverage of the bones is possible without tension at the closure of the wound.
- The preoperative TcPO2-measurement of the distal limb helps to define the level of amputation, on which wound healing can be expected.[46,47]
- Postoperative treatment consists always in the confection of an rTCC (*picture by Waibel and Boeni Chapter Charcot foot*), which allows the patient to ambulate with full weight bearing and protects the wound perfectly until the healing—which takes in diabetic patients often longer than in the normal patient population—is completed. Depending on the leg length discrepancy after the surgery, the patients need to wear height compensation on either side, to avoid problems with the balance or low back pain, as the protective postoperative cast may produce a functional leg length discrepancy.
- For auxiliary means, orthopedic shoe ware and loading analyses are performed in these patients, see also chapter "Charcot," by Waibel and Boeni[48–50]

SUMMARY

Mid- and hindfoot amputations are common treatment options in a patient with diabetic foot problems in order to avoid major amputations. Owing to the impaired vascular and neurologic situations in long-term diabetic patients, the hindfoot amputations are considered contra-indicated among experienced diabetic foot surgeons due to their high level of complications, most often ending in BKA. The main advantage of all the described surgeries is the option of ambulating short distances without an auxiliary device.

CLINICS CARE POINTS

- Perform preoperatively an analysis of the vascular and of the neurologic situation
- In case of doubt, amputate on a higher level in order to avoid revision surgery in these often polymorbid patients
- The surgeon must not only take care of the surgery and the follow up, but also of the correct fit of the orthotic or prosthetic device

DISCLOSURE

The author has nothing to disclose.

REFERENCES

1. Bertoni AG, Saydah S, Brancati FL. Diabetes and the risk of infection-related mortality in the U.S. Diabetes Care 2001;24(6):1044–9.
2. Gautieri A, Passini FS, Silvan U, et al. Advanced glycation end-products: Mechanics of aged collagen from molecule to tissue. Matrix Biol 2017;59:95–108.
3. Shah BR, Hux JE. Quantifying the risk of infectious diseases for people with diabetes. Diabetes Care 2003;26(2):510–3.
4. Bowker JH, San Giovanni TP. Amputations and disarticulations. Philadelphia: WB Saunders; 2000.
5. Bowker JH. Atlas of amputations and limb deficiencies. 3rd edition. Rosemont: AAOS; 2003.
6. Brown ML, Tang W, Patel A, et al. Partial foot amputation in patients with diabetic foot ulcers. Foot Ankle Int 2012;33(9):707–16.
7. Thorud JC, Jupiter DC, Lorenzana J, et al. Reoperation and reamputation after transmetatarsal amputation: a systematic review and meta-analysis. J Foot Ankle Surg 2016;55(5):1007–12.
8. Czerniecki JM, Turner AP, Williams RM, et al. The development and validation of the AMPREDICT model for predicting mobility outcome after dysvascular lower extremity amputation. J Vasc Surg 2017;65(1):162–171 e3.
9. Belon HP, Vigoda DF. Emotional adaptation to limb loss. Phys Med Rehabil Clin N Am 2014;25(1):53–74.
10. Baumgartner RA, Botta P. Amputation und Prothesenversorgung. 3rd edition. Stuttgart: Thieme; 2007.
11. Dillon MP, Barker TM. Comparison of gait of persons with partial foot amputation wearing prosthesis to matched control group: an observational study. J Rehabil Res Dev 2008;45(9):1317–34.
12. Esquenazi A. Gait analysis in lower-limb amputation and prosthetic rehabilitation. Phys Med Rehabil Clin N Am 2014;25(1):153–67.
13. Waters RL, Mulroy S. The energy expenditure of normal and pathologic gait. Gait Posture 1999;9(3):207–31.
14. Waters RL, Perry J, Antonelli D, et al. Energy cost of walking of amputees: the influence of level of amputation. J Bone Joint Surg Am 1976;58(1):42–6.
15. Schaefer MBT. Prosthetic fitting following amputations on the foot. FussSprungg 2019;17:155–70.
16. Baumgartner R. [Forefoot and midfoot amputations]. Oper Orthop Traumatol 2011;23(4):254–64.
17. DeCotiis MA. Lisfranc and Chopart amputations. Clin Podiatr Med Surg 2005; 22(3):385–93 [Review].
18. Elsharawy MA. Outcome of midfoot amputations in diabetic gangrene. Ann Vasc Surg 2011;25(6):778–82.
19. Stone PA, Back MR, Armstrong PA, et al. Midfoot amputations expand limb salvage rates for diabetic foot infections. Ann Vasc Surg 2005;19(6):805–11.
20. Lafiteau M. Observation sur une amputation partielle du pied. In: Lafiteau M, editor. La médecine éclairée par les sciences physique. Paris: Buisson; 1792. p. 85–8.
21. Lisfranc JM. Nouvelle methode opératoire pour l'amputation partielle dans son articulation tarso-metatarsienne. Paris: Sabon; 1815.
22. Roach JJ, Deutsch A, McFarlane DS. Resurrection of the amputations of Lisfranc and Chopart for diabetic gangrene. Arch Surg 1987;122(8):931–4.

23. Early JS. Transmetatarsal and midfoot amputations. Clin Orthop Relat Res 1999;(361):85–90.
24. Lieberman JR, Jacobs RL, Goldstock L, et al. Chopart amputation with percutaneous heel cord lengthening. Clin Orthop Relat Res 1993;(296):86–91.
25. Greene CJ, Bibbo C. The Lisfranc Amputation: a more reliable level of amputation with proper intraoperative tendon balancing. J Foot Ankle Surg 2017;56(4):824–6.
26. Hoke M. An operation for the correction of extremely relaxed flat feet. JBJS 1931; 13(4):773–83.
27. Sanders LJ. Transmetatarsal and midfoot amputations. Clin Podiatr Med Surg 1997;14(4):741–62.
28. Brodell JD Jr, Ayers BC, Baumhauer JF, et al. Chopart Amputation: questioning the clinical efficacy of a long-standing surgical option for diabetic foot infection. J Am Acad Orthop Surg 2020;28(16):684–91.
29. Green CJ, Bibbo C, McArdle A, et al. A functional Chopart's Amputation with tendon transfers. J Foot Ankle Surg 2021;60(1):213–7.
30. Faglia E, Clerici G, Frykberg R, et al. Outcomes of Chopart Amputation in a tertiary referral diabetic foot clinic: data from a consecutive series of 83 hospitalized patients. J Foot Ankle Surg 2016;55(2):230–4.
31. Krause FG, Pfander G, Henning J, et al. Ankle dorsiflexion arthrodesis to salvage Chopart's amputation with anterior skin insufficiency. Foot Ankle Int 2013;34(11): 1560–8.
32. Schade VL, Roukis TS, Yan JL. Factors associated with successful Chopart Amputation in patients with diabetes:a systematic review. Foot & Ankle Specialist 2010;3(5):278–84.
33. Taylor GI, Palmer JH. The vascular territories (angiosomes) of the body: experimental study and clinical applications. Br J Plast Surg 1987;40(2):113–41.
34. Rammelt S, Olbrich A, Zwipp H. [Hindfoot amputations]. Oper Orthop Traumatol 2011;23(4):265–79.
35. Strayer LM Jr. Recession of the gastrocnemius; an operation to relieve spastic contracture of the calf muscles. J Bone Joint Surg Am 1950;32-a(3):671–6.
36. Altindas M, Kilic A. Is Boyd's operation a last solution that may prevent major amputations in diabetic foot patients? J Foot Ankle Surg 2008;47(4):307–12.
37. Pirogoff NI. Resection of bones and joints and amputations and disarticulations of joints. Clin Orthop Relat Res 1864;1991(266):3–11.
38. Andronic O, Boeni T, Burkhard MD, et al. Modifications of the Pirogoff amputation technique in adults: A retrospective analysis of 123 cases. J Orthop 2020; 18:5–12.
39. Taniguchi A, Tanaka Y, Kadono K, et al. Pirogoff ankle disarticulation as an option for ankle disarticulation. Clin Orthop Relat Res 2003;414:322–8.
40. Kinner B, Roll C. [Modified Pirogoff's amputation]. Oper Orthop Traumatol 2016; 28(5):335–44.
41. Braaksma R, Dijkstra PU, Geertzen JHB. Syme Amputation: a systematic review. Foot Ankle Int 2018;39(3):284–91.
42. Syme J. Surgical cases and observations. Amputation at the ankle-joint. 1843. Clin Orthop Relat Res 1990;(256):3–6.
43. Finkler ES, Marchwiany DA, Schiff AP, et al. Long-term outcomes following Syme's Amputation. Foot Ankle Int 2017;38(7):732–5.
44. Schnur D, Meier RH 3rd. Amputation surgery. Phys Med Rehabil Clin N Am 2014; 25(1):35–43.
45. Garwood CS, Steinberg JS. Soft tissue balancing after partial foot amputations. Clin Podiatr Med Surg 2016;33(1):99–111.

46. Arsenault KA, Al-Otaibi A, Devereaux PJ, et al. The use of transcutaneous oximetry to predict healing complications of lower limb amputations: a systematic review and meta-analysis. Eur J Vasc Endovasc Surg 2012;43(3):329–36.

47. Berli MC, Wanivenhaus F, Kabelitz M, et al. Predictors for reoperation after lower limb amputation in patients with peripheral arterial disease. Vasa 2019;48(5):419–24.

48. Kaib T, Block J, Heitzmann DWW, et al. Prosthetic restoration of the forefoot lever after Chopart amputation and its consequences onto the limb during gait. Gait Posture 2019;73:1–7.

49. Krause FG, Aebi H, Lehmann O, et al. The "flap-shaft" prosthesis for insensate feet with Chopart or Lisfranc amputations. Foot Ankle Int 2007;28(2):255–62.

50. Philbin TM, Leyes M, Sferra JJ, et al. Orthotic and prosthetic devices in partial foot amputations. Foot Ankle Clin 2001;6(2):215–28, v.

Moving?

Make sure your subscription moves with you!

To notify us of your new address, find your **Clinics Account Number** (located on your mailing label above your name), and contact customer service at:

Email: journalscustomerservice-usa@elsevier.com

800-654-2452 (subscribers in the U.S. & Canada)
314-447-8871 (subscribers outside of the U.S. & Canada)

Fax number: 314-447-8029

Elsevier Health Sciences Division
Subscription Customer Service
3251 Riverport Lane
Maryland Heights, MO 63043

*To ensure uninterrupted delivery of your subscription, please notify us at least 4 weeks in advance of move.

ELSEVIER

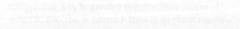

Printed and bound by CPI Group (UK) Ltd, Croydon, CR0 4YY

08/05/2025

01864715-0004